Bloody Bioethics

This is the first book to argue in favor of paying people for their blood plasma. It does not merely argue that offering compensation to plasma donors is morally permissible. It argues that prohibiting donor compensation is morally *wrong* – and that it is morally wrong for all of the reasons that are offered against allowing donor compensation.

Opponents of donor compensation claim that it will reduce the amount and quality of plasma obtained, exploit and coerce donors, and undermine social cohesion. James Stacey Taylor argues that empirical evidence demonstrates that compensating plasma donors greatly increases the amount of plasma obtained with no adverse effects on the quality of the pharmaceutical products that are manufactured from it. Prohibiting compensation thus harms patients by reducing their access to the medicines they need. He also argues that it is the prohibition of compensation – not its offer – that exploits donors, fails to respect the moral need to secure a person's authoritative consent to her treatment, and prevents donors from giving their informed consent to donate. Prohibiting compensation thus not only harms patients but also wrongs donors.

Bloody Bioethics will appeal to researchers, advanced students, and medical professionals interested in bioethics, moral philosophy, and the moral limits of markets.

James Stacey Taylor is Professor of Philosophy at The College of New Jersey, USA. He is the author of *Death, Posthumous Harm, and Bioethics* (2012), *Practical Autonomy and Bioethics* (2009), *Stakes and Kidneys: Why Markets in Human Body Parts are Morally Imperative* (2005), and *Markets with Limits* (2022). He is the editor of *The Metaphysics and Ethics of Death: New Essays* (2013) and *Personal Autonomy: New Essays on Personal Autonomy and Its Role in Contemporary Moral Philosophy* (2005).

Routledge Annals of Bioethics

Series Editors:
Mark J. Cherry

For more information about this series, please visit: www.routledge.com/Routledge-Annals-of-Bioethics/book-series/RAB

Bloody Bioethics
Why Prohibiting Plasma Compensation Harms Patients and Wrongs Donors

James Stacey Taylor

Routledge
Taylor & Francis Group

NEW YORK AND LONDON

First published 2022
by Routledge
605 Third Avenue, New York, NY 10158

and by Routledge
4 Park Square, Milton Park, Abingdon, Oxon, OX14 4RN

Routledge is an imprint of the Taylor & Francis Group, an informa business

Library of Congress Cataloging-in-Publication Data
A catalog record for this title has been requested

ISBN: 978-1-032-20386-7 (hbk)
ISBN: 978-1-032-20505-2 (pbk)
ISBN: 978-1-003-26391-3 (ebk)

DOI: 10.4324/9781003263913

Typeset in Sabon
by Apex CoVantage, LLC

This volume is dedicated to all the patients across the world who need plasma or plasma-derived medical products.

It is also dedicated to all the plasma donors who give of themselves to aid them, the dedicated healthcare professionals who care for them, those who serve them by protecting their interests, and everyone in the industry associated with the sourcing of plasma and the manufacture of plasma-derived medicinal products – whether commercial or otherwise.

Contents

Acknowledgments

This volume would not exist had Sally Satel not introduced me to Josh Penrod. I am thus very grateful to Sally for this introduction – as well as for being interested in my earlier work on kidney markets and noting its relevance to the related issue of donor compensation.

As a result of Sally's introduction, I have incurred numerous debts of gratitude to people involved with the donation of plasma, its manufacture into plasma-derived medicinal products, and the patient use of these products – as well as to many, many patients. My first debt here is to Josh Penrod, Jan Bult, and Joe Rosen. As leading members of the Plasma Protein Therapeutics Association (PPTA), they took the chance that an academic philosopher might have something useful to contribute to the discussion about the ethics of donor compensation. I am deeply grateful to them for this, and for their friendship and guidance over the past several years. I also thank the PPTA for the many opportunities that they have given me to present earlier versions of many sections of this volume at various professional events attended by persons associated with the collection of plasma for use by patients. The comments and criticisms that I received on those occasions were invariably helpful – and sometimes trenchant! – and have helped me make this volume be far better than it would otherwise have been.

I am also grateful to Jose Drabwell, Saara Kiema, Magda Lourenco, Nizar Mahlaoui, Julia Nordin, Martine Pergent, Johan Prevot, John Seymour, Leire Solis, and Martin Van Hagen of the International Patient Organisation for Primary Immunodeficiencies (IPOPI) for their support, encouragement, extremely helpful discussions of my work, and for their tireless work to support the interests of patients. I also thank IPOPI for generously extending to me speaking invitations to discuss ethical issues associated with the care of patients with primary immunodeficiencies (PIDs) – and I thank all of the members of IPOPI for their work on behalf of patients. I similarly thank Carla Duff, Geraldine Dunne, Rosalind Fisher, Dorothea Grosse-Kreul, Karen Henderson, and Karin Ludwig of the International Nursing Group for Immunodeficiencies (INGID) for their insights into the ethical issues associated with the care of patients with PID and for their ceaseless work on their behalf. I thank INGID too for their generous speaking invitations to discuss ethical issues associated with the care of patients with PID – and I thank all of the members of INGID for the care and support that they provide to their patients.

My work on the ethics of donor compensation has greatly benefitted from discussions with many people. I especially thank Sonia Balboni, Julie Birkofer, Roger Brinser, Jan Bult, Rose Bult, Mark J. Cherry, John K. Davis, John Delacourt, William English, Nahla Erwa, Julia Fabens, Albert Farrugia, Alain Fischer, Randy Furby, Peter Jaworski, Bobby Gaspar, Jason Grinnell, Mary Gustafson, Larry Hall, Steven Holland, Nicola Lacetera, Bruce Lim, Mario Macis, Tom May, Dominika Misztela, Joe Rosen, Kurt Rotthoff, George Schreiber, Jeremy Shearmur, Bill Speir, James Spence, Bobbi Stackman, Paul W. Strengers, Margaret Taylor-Ulizio, Paul Tudico, Mirjam van der Burg, Shinji Wada, and Alexa Wetzel for their helpful comments as this project progressed.

I also thank Josh Penrod and Julia Fabens for their extremely generous and helpful written comments on Chapter 1, and Francoise Rossi for her incisive questions about my account of exploitation which afforded me the opportunity better to express my views.

Parts of this volume have been presented at the Plasma Protein Therapeutics Association Business Forum (in 2018 and 2019), California State University at Fullerton, Georgetown University, the Columbia Economics Club of Columbia South Carolina, Towson University, Adrian College, the 2016 International Plasma Protein Congress, and the 2013 Plasma Protein Therapeutics Association Annual Meeting. I thank my audiences on those occasions for their insightful comments and criticisms.

I am also *very* grateful to the Institute for Humane Studies for hosting a workshop in 2020 on an earlier draft of this volume. I thank Stewart Robertson and Adrienne DePrisco for organizing the workshop and all of those who participated in it – Andrew I. Cohen, David Dick, Iskra Fileva, Bill Glod, Michael Huemer, Peter Jaworski, Nancy Jecker, Chris MacDonald, Mario Macis, Vida Panitch, Travis Timmerman, Christopher Tollefsen, Jeppe von Platz, and Steven Weimer – for their very helpful comments and suggestions.

Given the conclusions that I reach in this volume, I should stress even more than usual that the views expressed here are mine, and mine alone!

I also thank Mark J. Cherry and Ana Iltis for their support and encouragement during the completion of this project, and the referees who reviewed it for the Annals of Bioethics for their excellent – and very helpful – comments. I thank, too, Andrew Weckenmann and Allie Simmons and of Routledge for their support; I especially thank Andrew for his sage advice on the title.

This project was completed during a semester-long sabbatical from The College of New Jersey. I thank the College for providing me with this time to write. I also thank the staff of the R. Barbara Gitenstein

Library at The College of New Jersey for their work in fulfilling my many Interlibrary Loan requests.

An earlier version of Chapter 2 appeared as "Why Prohibiting Donor Compensation Can Prevent Plasma Donors From Giving Their Informed Consent to Donate," *Journal of Medicine and Philosophy*, 44, 1 (2019): 10–32. I thank the Editor of that journal, Mark J. Cherry, for permission to reprint here. Sections of the Conclusion initially appeared in "Why Policies That Aim at National Self-Sufficiency in Blood and Blood Products Are (Usually) Unethical," *Public Affairs Quarterly*, 29, 3 (2015): 313–326. I thank the Editor of that journal, Nicholas Rescher, for permission to reprint here. I also thank the referees of those earlier papers for their exceptionally helpful comments on them.

Preface

This is a work of moral philosophy. But despite my academic approach the topic that I am addressing – the ethics of offering financial compensation to prospective plasma donors – is of critical practical import. Around 6 million people globally are affected by primary immunodeficiencies, with a further c. 1.125 million men being affected by hemophilia.[1] Plasma is needed to produce the pharmaceuticals that these people need. If not enough is secured to meet their medical needs they will suffer, and, in some cases, die. The only way to secure enough plasma to meet the medical needs of patients is to offer compensation to prospective donors.

In an ideal world, the last four sentences of the previous paragraph would suffice to establish that plasma donors should be compensated, and this volume would be unnecessary. But we do not live in an ideal world. As a result of the widespread and unjust prohibition of donor compensation, patients needlessly continue to suffer and die.

Why is this so? Being as charitable as possible it appears that those who oppose donor compensation are not primarily concerned about the effects that allowing it would have on patients. The evidence is overwhelming that when current best practices are followed compensated donation increases the amount of plasma secured with no decrease in the quality of the medicinal products that are manufactured from it. (Although these facts do not prevent some opponents of donor compensation from continuing to argue that offering compensation will reduce the amount of plasma secured and lower its quality.) It thus appears that those who oppose compensation are concerned with the effects that this would have on donors. They express concern that (for example) offers of compensation would exploit donors or lead to their economic situations coercing them into donating. I argue in this volume that not only are these concerns mistaken but that they backfire: It is the *prohibition* of compensation that subjects donors to (for example) exploitation and coercion. I hope that showing this will help change the minds of those who currently oppose allowing compensation to be offered to plasma donors out of concern for them, paving the way for compensation to be allowed, so that patients will have greater access to the plasma-based treatments that they so desperately need.

I first became interested in the ethics of offering compensation to prospective plasma donors in 2013. At that time, Sally Satel introduced me to Joshua Penrod, the Vice President of a division of Plasma Protein Therapeutics Association (PPTA), the trade association representing the manufacturers of human plasma protein therapies and the collectors of human plasma. Josh was interested in talking with me and other scholars about ethical issues associated with plasma collection, from both compensated and uncompensated donors.

Sally introduced me to Josh as she knew of my work defending markets in kidneys for transplant and thought that I would be interested in becoming better acquainted with the arguments surrounding the ethics of offering compensation to prospective plasma donors. At the time I thought that any debate over compensating plasma donors would be philosophically uninteresting. Unlike kidneys, plasma is renewable, the amounts offered to encourage persons to donate are relatively small, and the risks to donors are negligible. I could see no ethical problems at all with offering plasma donors compensation. But the opportunity for an excursion outside the ivory tower was appealing, and so I met with Josh and Joe Rosen (the former Chairman of PPTA). As a result of this meeting, Josh invited me both to visit a plasma center in Maryland to see how they operate and to give a talk at the PPTA Annual Meeting in Denver.

Since I believed that it was obvious that offering compensation to plasma donors was ethically permissible, I had to give a lot of thought to come up with a talk that would be at least moderately interesting to people in the industry. At the time I was preparing to teach a class on the moral limits of markets which included discussion on the role that prices play as signaling mechanisms. This led me to realize that offers of compensation could function similarly, and so my talk (which was a very early ancestor of Chapter 2 of this volume) focused on the ethical need to offer compensation to prospective donors to secure their informed consent to donate.

Once I realized that the moral concern with securing donors' informed consent to donate required that offers of compensation be available to them, I began to wonder whether other moral concerns expressed about the treatment of donors would similarly support the need to offer compensation. I explored this idea in a series of talks given to various audiences associated with the plasma industry, including PPTA, regulators, healthcare professionals devoted to the care of patients who needed plasma-based therapies, and organizations focused on advocating for the interests of patients. I learned so much from these interactions, including (importantly) how to situate my philosophical arguments so that they were directly applicable to the policy debates that affected patients' lives. Most importantly, I was forcibly struck – time and time and time again – by the terrible human cost that must be paid by patients and those who love them and care for them when the plasma-based therapies that they need are rendered inaccessible to them by the decisions of bureaucrats.

As I noted earlier, this is a work of moral philosophy. The conclusions that I draw in this volume – that prohibiting compensation to plasma donors wrongs and harms patients, and wrongs donors – are thus the result of the arguments that I offer. This should go without saying but I mention it here for two reasons. First, I observed earlier that it seemed obvious to me that plasma donors should receive compensation. This might give rise to the suspicion that I had already settled on my conclusions prior to engaging with the arguments and writing this volume. But while I initially believed that plasma donors should be compensated the conclusions that the arguments in this volume have led me to endorse are distinct from (and far stronger than) my original view. My original view was merely that plasma donors should be compensated. Now, not only do I believe this to be the case but I also believe that the moral concerns about donors (e.g., that they be free from coercion or exploitation) that are offered to justify the prohibition of donor compensation instead require that it be allowed. Second, I have sometimes been asked (rather pointedly) how much of an honorarium I have received to speak in favor of donor compensation. The answer has always been simple: Nothing. While (most of) my travel expenses have been paid by the organizations that have invited me to speak, I have never accepted an honorarium for doing so. The sole exception to this was when I accepted an honorarium from a pharmaceutical company to speak on "Ethical Issues in Nursing" at a conference in Amsterdam – a presentation that had nothing to do with plasma. The arguments in this volume are thus unsullied by fiscal interest – although they are not similarly detached from a concern for the interests of patients.

Note

1. Isabelle Meyts et al., "Primary Immunodeficiencies: A Decade of Progress and a Promising Future," *Frontiers in Immunology* 11 (2021), 1; Alfonso Iorio, Jeffrey S. Stonebraker, Hervé Chambost, Michael Makris, Donna Coffin, Christine Herr, and Federico Germini, "Establishing the Prevalence and Prevalence at Birth of Hemophilia in Males: A Meta-analytic Approach Using National Registries," *Annals of Internal Medicine* 171, 8 (2019), 542.

Introduction

The debate over the ethics of compensating the donors of blood and blood products has now settled into a familiar pattern. Those who object to this practice hold that offering donors compensation will adversely affect the interests of patients who need blood and blood products by jeopardizing the safety of their supply and diminishing the amounts that are collected. These empirical claims are then supported by two moral claims that are ostensibly intended to protect donors. First, that offering compensation will be a wrongful proposal for it will undermine donors' autonomy by enabling them to be coerced into donating by their economic situation. Second, that compensated donors will be exploited by the commercial plasma centers to which they donate. These concerns for donors and patients are then buttressed with the claim that offering donors compensation could adversely affect the interests of everyone in the society in which this occurs through undermining social cohesion. In response to these objections, those who defend compensated donation argue that none of these claims are true. In this "stately scholastic minuet," the opponents of donor compensation lead while its defenders follow.[1]

It is time for those who support compensating plasma donors to reverse this dance and go on the offensive.

But this is not a mere *scholastic* minuet of only academic interest. The question of whether plasma donors should be compensated is of critical practical import. Most obviously, this is because the prohibition of donor compensation – a prohibition that is often supported by appeal to moral argument – *harms patients* by making the critical medications that they need less accessible to them. Prohibiting compensation also wrongs some donors. It precludes them from being able to give their informed consent to their donation, renders them vulnerable to impermissible offers, and subjects them to exploitation. None of these are trivial concerns. Indeed, it is not an exaggeration to say that for many patients getting the conclusion of this debate right and allowing donors to be compensated is a matter of life or death. The current academic and political preference for

DOI: 10.4324/9781003263913-1

prohibiting donor compensation means that this debate is less of a stately scholarly minuet than it is a *danse macabre*.

The Focus of This Volume: Financial Compensation for Plasma Donation

In this volume, I focus on establishing the ethical necessity of *financially* compensating plasma donors. Other types of incentive that are offered to plasma donors – such as paid days off work, raffle tickets for big-ticket prizes, scholarships paid directly to academic institutions, and nontransferable gift cards – appear not to concern most of the opponents of compensated donation who do not consider them to be "compensation."[2] I will assume for the sake of argument that there is a morally relevant difference somewhere in this apparently "absurd" distinction and that financial compensation is somehow morally distinct from the other valuable goods that are offered to donors.[3]

Plasma is a straw-colored liquid in which blood cells are suspended. It is "an aqueous solution of various inorganic salts . . . with a high concentration of various proteins (plasma derivatives)."[4] Plasma is obtained either from whole blood donated for transfusion purposes or through plasmapheresis from donors in plasma collection centers. (Plasmapheresis is a process that separates the blood cells from the liquid plasma and returns the cells to the donor.[5]) Plasma that is obtained from whole blood donation is termed "recovered plasma" and is 10–15% of the plasma secured.[6] Recovered plasma can be used as fresh frozen plasma (FFP), convalescent plasma therapy (CPT), or as raw material for the manufacture of plasma-derived medicinal products (PDMPs).[7] Plasma obtained directly from plasma donors is termed "source plasma" and provides 85–90% of plasma secured.[8] Source plasma from compensated donors is used exclusively for the manufacture of PDMPs. Over 1,000 plasma donations are needed to manufacture a single PDMP – and so given the demand for PDMPs the need for plasma is significant.[9] Part of the process of manufacturing PDMP involves fractionation, in which the plasma proteins are separated into "fractions of more or less purified proteins with different properties."[10] The manufacturing process allows for the identification and elimination of known pathogens that might have contaminated the source plasma.[11] PDMPs include clotting factor concentrates F VIII and F IX, immunoglobulins, and hyperimmune globulins (rabies, hepatitis B, RhIG). They are often infused or injected into persons who have missing or deficient proteins.[12] The diseases or conditions that they treat are typically rare, and include hemophilia A, hemophilia B,[13] Von Willebrand Disease,[14] and many primary immunodeficiency diseases.[15] PDMPs are also used to treat burn victims.[16] More recently, PDMPs have been proposed for the treatment of COVID-19.[17] Several PDMPs (including anti-D immunoglobulin, anti-rabies immunoglobulin, anti-tetanus immunoglobulin, coagulation factor VIII, and coagulation factor IX) are listed on the World Health Organization's Model List of Essential Medicines (EML).[18] Indeed, plasma is of such medical importance that it should be considered a strategic resource.[19]

I focus on the ethical necessity of compensating plasma donors for three reasons.

First, to put things bluntly, plasma is where the action is.[20] There is currently a tension between the increasing world demand for PDMPs and the internationally dominant policy position that prohibits donor compensation. This tension must be resolved. The world demand for PDMPs is likely to grow. Many patients currently do not receive the medical care that they need owing to its cost. As Paul F.W. Strengers notes, "only 30% of the patients with hemophilia A or B have been diagnosed and only 25% receive treatment."[21] The International Patient Organisation for Primary Immunodeficiencies (IPOPI) observes that worldwide less than 10% of patients with primary immunodeficiency diseases (PID) are diagnosed and only 6% receive treatment with immunoglobulin.[22] These dire numbers could improve as increasing incomes across the globe are likely to lead to improvement in medical care. (This is a consummation *devoutly* to be wished, especially for patients with hemophilia or PID.) This could lead to increased patient demand for PDMPs both as a result of an increased ability to afford appropriate medication and as a result of improved diagnostic capabilities. There is also currently considerable research into the development of new treatments for disorders (e.g., Alzheimer's disease) that draw on plasma proteins, which, if successful, will further stimulate demand for PDMPs.[23] And, as noted earlier, plasma is also being utilized in new therapies for COVID-19.[24]

But as things stand, this increasing demand is likely to go unmet – to the detriment of patients. Although (as I will establish in Chapter 1) compensated donation is necessary to secure a sufficient amount of plasma to meet medical demand, the dominant policy throughout the world favors its prohibition. The World Health Organization (WHO), for example, has been vocal in its opposition to compensating the donors of blood and blood products. And – as is to be expected – its expressed concerns follow the established steps of the "stately scholastic minuet" that is the current debate over donor compensation. The WHO expresses concern with the safety of the supply of blood and blood products, voices the fear that the offers of compensation could be so "tantalizing" to prospective donors that they would be unable to genuinely consent to donate,[25] and worries that donors will be exploited.[26] As a result it supports eliminating all compensation paid to donors. This position – expressed most clearly in its 2013 publication *Towards Self-Sufficiency in Safe Blood and Blood Products based on Voluntary Non-remunerated Donation* – is most definitely *not* merely a scholastic one. It has garnered "the support of Ministries of Health in 51 countries from all regions of the world" and was influential in motivating the provincial government of Ontario, Canada, to enact legislation that banned compensation for blood or plasma donation.[27] In 2017, Alberta followed Ontario in banning compensation for blood or plasma donation.[28] (This ban was reversed by the Voluntary Blood Donations Repeal Act of 2020.)[29] British Columbia banned offers of compensation in 2018.[30] Quebec banned offers of compensation for blood and plasma in 1994.[31]

The widespread prohibition of making offers of compensation to plasma donors might be explained in part by the fact that unlike donors of many other bodily parts or services plasma donors have a long history of receiving financial compensation for their services. The donors of many other bodily goods and services are either uncompensated (e.g., whole blood donors and – with the exception of Iran – kidney donors)[32] or the goods or services that they provide (e.g., surrogate pregnancy, bone marrow) do not have an extensive history of being legally procurable for compensation.[33] This history might explain why the commercial collection of plasma is the focus of those who oppose the offer of compensation for bodily goods and services for medical purposes. If one believes that offers of compensation to secure bodily parts or services are wrongful, one will be more likely to focus one's efforts on working to remove those offers that are currently being made rather than on opposing offers that are already prohibited. This focus on eliminating those offers of compensation that are currently being made to prospective plasma donors might also be motivated in part by a visceral objection to what is perceived to be the commercial plasma industry's profitability.[34] And – as I will note in Chapter 6 – some groups might have a vested economic interest in opposing donor compensation.

Whatever the explanation (or explanations) for the widespread prohibition on offering prospective plasma donors compensation, it is highly unfortunate for it limits the availability of plasma and in doing so harms the patients who need it. To ensure that PDMPs are accessible to the increasing numbers of patients who need them and who would be able to secure them if they were available, it is important to demonstrate that the ethical objections to donor compensation are unfounded. Achieving this should – when combined with a concern for the well-being of patients – pave the way to revoking the legal prohibitions on compensated donation. And since it can also be shown that the prohibition of donor compensation should be condemned by the same ethical considerations that are mistakenly invoked to support it, this patient-focused impetus to allow donor compensation will *also* be supported by a moral concern for donors.

Second, in addition to being where "the action" is, the debate over the compensation of plasma donors is more purely a debate over *ethics* than are similar debates over the morality of compensating the donors of other bodily parts or services. Debates over whether persons should receive compensation for their bodily parts or services need to address two related issues. They need to address questions concerning the effects that offers of compensation would have on both the quality and the quantity of the goods or services in question that are procured. They also need to address questions concerning the effects that the provision of compensation will have on the persons to whom this is offered. They need to ask, for example, whether the offer of compensation will lead to the exploitation or coercion of donors. The first set of questions might be called the *instrumental* questions about the effects of allowing compensation to be offered; the second might be called the *normative* questions that could (and should) be raised about this.[35] Given that compensation for many bodily goods and services is either prohibited or has only recently been legally permitted answers to the questions of what effects the provision of compensation would have on both the quality and quantity of the goods or services in question often have limited empirical support.[36] By contrast, the effects that compensating plasma donors has on both the quantity of the plasma secured and the quality of the PDMPs that are produced from it are well known. Compensating plasma donors results in a far *greater* amount of plasma being procured with *no* adverse effects on the safety of the PDMPs that this plasma is used to produce. Objections to compensated donation thus cannot be based on concerns about the instrumental effects of compensation.[37] The objections to this practice must thus focus on the normative questions that it raises.

Third, I focus on the ethical need to compensate plasma donors in this volume because the policy of many countries toward plasma procurement appears to be bizarre in a way that their policies toward the procurement of other bodily goods and services do not. Many countries prohibit offering compensation to domestic plasma donors. This often (if not always) leads to a shortfall in the amount of plasma that they obtain relative to the medical needs of their populace. Many then make up this shortfall by importing plasma from countries that they know obtained it through donor compensation. This is striking – and apparently bizarre. If the prohibition of donor compensation is justified on either instrumental or moral grounds (e.g., plasma from compensated donors puts patients at risk, or it exploits donors) then it would seem that these grounds would support not only a refusal to allow donor compensation domestically but also a refusal to encourage this practice abroad. (If the use of plasma from compensated donors really does put patients at risk, then this would give reason to avoid it whether it was obtained from domestic or foreign donors.) This differential treatment of domestic and foreign donors does not occur with respect to other bodily goods (e.g., kidneys) or services (e.g., surrogate pregnancy). No country prohibits, for example, the compensation of domestic kidney donors and then imports transplant kidneys from abroad. I will explain in this volume why this differential treatment of domestic and foreign donors could be justified with plasma. I will then argue that this proposed justification is unsound.

Before providing an outline of my arguments in this volume, two further points should be noted. First, my arguments in support of the ethical necessity of compensating plasma donors are not immediately generalizable to the debates that concern compensating the donors of other bodily goods (such as kidneys or ova) or services (such as surrogate pregnancy). As I will discuss in the Conclusion to this volume, there are important differences between the donation of source plasma for processing into PDMPs and the donation of other bodily goods or services (such as whole blood, kidneys, bone marrow, ova, or surrogate pregnancy). For my arguments in this volume to be applied to the question of whether the donors of other bodily parts or services should be compensated for their donations, the relevant differences between plasma and the other bodily parts or services at issue would need to be recognized and (if necessary) my arguments adjusted to accommodate these differences. (This volume should thus be understood as a complement to, but not an extension of, my earlier work on the morality of markets in human transplant kidneys.)[38] The focus of *Bloody Bioethics* is on plasma, and plasma alone. Second, as T.M. Wilkinson has noted in the context of the debates over whether human transplant organs should be bought and sold on the marketplace, the opponents of compensation "have been much less thorough in setting out their case" than those who favor it.[39] As a result, "much of the case in favour of sale has involved setting out the details of what the case against ought to have said before trying to rebut it."[40] Those who oppose offering compensation to plasma donors have similarly failed to develop thorough arguments for their positions. Since this is not merely a scholastic debate but one that has critical implications for healthcare policy, it is more than usually important for its conclusions to be correct. To this end, I will not merely address the arguments of those who oppose donor compensation as these appear in the literature but will take care to develop the best version possible of each position that I criticize. (In some cases – such as in my discussion of social cohesion – this will require that I develop original arguments against donor compensation either to support conclusions that are either offered by those who oppose donor compensation or that should be offered by them given their theoretical commitments.) This will provide the best assurance possible that the conclusions arrived at in this volume are sound.

Should Donors Be Compensated? A Focus on Ethics

My arguments in *Bloody Bioethics* begin in Chapter 1 with an overview of the instrumental effects of donor compensation on both the overall amount of plasma obtained and the quality of the PDMPs that are manufactured from source plasma secured from compensated donors. I argue that the offer of financial compensation to donors neither compromises the safety of patients nor leads to a reduction in the amount of plasma collected – indeed, if donors are compensated at sufficient levels, this will *increase* the amount of plasma that is collected. This conclusion is compatible with the claim that some donors will be deterred from donating if donor compensation is allowed. (It is compatible because the number of donors who would only donate if compensation above a certain level is offered is greater than the number of donors who would only donate if compensation is not offered.) This claim is often offered as part of an argument against donor compensation that holds that it is possible that offers of donor compensation will reduce the overall amount of plasma collected. In Chapter 1, I will show that this argument is unsound. But I will accept that the claim that it is based on – that some donors will cease donating once compensation is offered – is true. I will, however, argue in Chapter 2 that not only does the argument that this observation is intended to support fail but that a reasonable explanation of why some donors cease to donate once compensation is offered supports the moral necessity of donor compensation. This explanation for the decrease in the number of persons who donate once low levels of compensation are offered is that the low level of compensation offered signals to donors that their donation is of lower value than they thought. This information leads them to decide not to donate. If this is true for some donors, then they would not have been able to give their informed consent to donate when the information contained in the offer of compensation was absent. To ensure that these donors are able to give their informed consent to donate compensation must thus be permitted. The use of the "crowding out" claim to oppose donor compensation thus backfires.

I then argue in Chapter 3 that the argument that offering donors compensation will compromise their autonomy with respect to their donations similarly backfires. Although this objection is widespread in both the academic and policy literature on donor compensation, it is rarely developed. To rectify this, I give aid and comfort to the opponents of donor compensation by developing an argument that establishes the central claim that the proponents of this objection endorse: That offers can function similarly to threats in diminishing the autonomy of those who accept them. But, I argue, this alone does not establish that offers of compensation are wrongful. To establish whether a proposal (whether classified as a threat or an offer) together with the exchange that occurs consequently upon it is wrongful, one must determine whether those who would be party to it would, given that it has been presented to them, *both* prefer to accept it rather than not *and* prefer that it be presented to them. If both conditions are met, then the proposal is permissible. However, if one or both of these conditions are *not* met, and the proposed transaction still occurs, then it would have occurred without the genuine consent of one of those party to it. The transaction would thus be wrongful. I will argue that while proposals of compensation are likely to meet both of these conditions proposals of penalties (i.e., those would be imposed in a regime that prohibited compensation) would not. The moral concern for donor autonomy thus both supports donor compensation and rejects its prohibition.

The importance not only of allowing compensation to be offered but allowing the level offered to reflect the relationship between the supply of plasma and the demand for it that informed the discussion in Chapter 2 also plays a role in Chapters 4 and 5 in the context of the claim that offers of compensation could exploit donors. In Chapter 4, I outline and defend an account of exploitation. Drawing on this account, I then argue in Chapter 5 that not only are the compensation levels that donors are currently offered not exploitative but that the prohibition of compensation could exploit some donors. I will then argue that some donors are exploited in countries when compensation is prohibited. The moral concern with avoiding exploitation thus requires that compensation be offered to donors.

By the end of Chapter 5, I would have established that the decision of some donors to cease donating once compensation is introduced shows that offers of compensation enable them to be better informed about their decisions and so is to be welcomed, that the offer of donor compensation would not be a proposal that could lead to a wrongful exchange, and that offers of compensation will not exploit donors. I would *also* have established that the *prohibition* of donor compensation would prevent some donors from being able to give their informed consent to donate, that this would constitute a wrongful proposal that could lead to a wrongful exchange (i.e., legislators refraining from prosecution in exchange for plasma centers and donors refraining from engaging in compensated donation), and that it enables some plasma centers that do not compensate their donors to exploit them.

At this juncture, the opponents of donor compensation will no longer be leading this scholarly minuet. Instead, they should be preparing to follow *my* lead. This is because at this point in the debate, I would have established that their position is morally wrong – and so unless they wish to abandon it, they must defend it.[41] To defend it they could (and, I will argue, to avoid a charge of hypocrisy *should*) argue that donor compensation should be prohibited on the grounds that even though this would both harm patients and wrong donors these harms and wrongs are outweighed by the moral importance of securing social cohesion through prohibiting donor compensation. This appeal to social cohesion could also be used to justify the common practice of prohibiting donor compensation domestically while importing plasma from abroad (e.g., from the United States) that is known to have been secured from compensated donors. In brief, the argument would be as follows: In *our* society, we ascribe a particular social meaning to uncompensated acts of donation and as a result these acts are necessary to cultivate and maintain the cohesiveness of our society. In *their* society, however, they might ascribe a different meaning to these actions, and so they are not (and should not be) as concerned to preserve the occurrence of uncompensated acts of donation to maintain the cohesiveness of their society.[42] Thus, while *we* should prohibit donor compensation to cultivate and maintain social cohesion, *they* do not need to do this. It is thus morally acceptable for us to import plasma (and PDMPs) from them even though we know that this has been secured (or they have been manufactured from plasma that has been secured) from compensated donors.

In Chapters 6 and 7, I work on behalf of those who oppose the compensation of domestic donors but who do not similarly oppose the importation of plasma from foreign donors they know to have been compensated to develop the most persuasive forms of this argument from social cohesion available. Alas, my work here will provide only cold comfort for the opponents of donor compensation for even the best forms of these arguments are unsound. There is thus no reason to oppose allowing plasma centers to offer compensation to their donors. This is especially so if one is willing to import plasma (and PDMPs) secured from compensated donors to meet the medical needs of one's population that would otherwise be medically underserved by one's own (uncompensated) procurement program.

In the Conclusion to this volume, I will expand the scope of my arguments beyond their prior focus on moral philosophy to engage with an aspect of the economics of plasma procurement: The question of from where countries should secure the plasma that is needed by the patients that reside within them. I will close by noting that my arguments in this volume will not necessarily translate into debates concerning the morality of compensating the donors of other bodily parts or services, such as kidneys, bone marrow, ova, semen, or surrogate pregnancy. They only establish that prohibiting the offer of compensation to prospective *plasma* donors harms patients and wrongs donors. And if this wrongful prohibition is (mistakenly) held to be justified on ethical grounds then that will be a bloody bioethics indeed.

Notes

1. The phrase "stately scholastic minuet" was used by Mary Warnock in her review of James Stacey Taylor, *Stakes and Kidneys: Why Markets in Human Body Parts are Morally Imperative* (Aldershot, UK: Ashgate, 2005). See her "Will Liberty Lead Us to an Internal Market?" *The Times Higher Education Supplement* (April 7, 2006). Available at: www.timeshighereducation.com/books/will-liberty-lead-us-to-an-internal-market/202438.article. I respond to Warnock's criticisms in "Kidney problems," *The Times Higher Education Supplement* (April 14, 2006). Available at: www.timeshighereducation.com/comment/letters/kidney-problems/202593.article

2. Joshua Penrod and Albert Farrugia noted that "while compensated plasma donors are . . . generally held in disdain for 'donating for the cash,' . . . ostensibly noncompensated blood donors are rewarded with chances at winning a television set, gift cards to a furniture store . . . tickets to the SuperBowl . . . tickets for admission to the zoo . . . and even a chance at a new car . . . This is clearly an absurd situation." "Errors and Omissions: Donor Compensation Policies and Richard Titmuss," *HEC Forum* 27, 4 (2015), 322. Similar skepticism was earlier expressed by A.A. Farrugia, J. Penrod, and J.M. Bult in "Payment, Compensation and Replacement – the Ethics and Motivation of Blood and Plasma Donation," *Vox Sanguinis* 60, S3 (2010), 205–206. See also Beth H. Shaz, Ronald E. Domen, and Christopher R. France, "Remunerating Donors to Ensure a Safe and Available Blood Supply," *Transfusion* 60, S3 (2020), S135. Shaz et al. refer to the gifts offered to blood donors that are considered not to constitute compensation for donation, but their skepticism can be generalized to similar putatively non-compensatory gifts offered to plasma donors. I outline a possible way to distinguish financial compensation from other valuable goods offered to donors in Chapter 3.
3. The absurdity of this distinction was noted by Penrod and Farrugia in "Errors and Omissions," 322.
4. Piet J. Hagen, *Blood Transfusion in Europe: A "White Paper"* (Strasbourg: Council of Europe Press, 1993), 190.
5. Ibid.
6. Jan Hartmann and Harvey G. Klein, "Supply and Demand for Plasma-Derived Medicinal Products - A Critical Reassessment Amid the COVID-19 Pandemic," *Transfusion* 60, 11 (2020), 2748.
7. Johan Prevot and Stephen Jolles, "Global Immunoglobulin Supply: Steaming Towards the Iceberg?" *Current Opinion in Allergy and Clinical Immunology* 20, 6 (2020), 557–558.
8. Hartmann and Klein, "Supply and Demand," 2748.
9. Paul F.W. Strengers, "Evidence-Based Clinical Indications of Plasma Products and Future Prospects," *Annals of Blood* 2, 9 (2017), 1. As many as 1,200 donations can be needed to treat just one patient for one year for hemophilia. See Tomasz Kluszczynski, Silvia Rohr, and Rianne Ernst, *White Paper: Key Economic and Value Considerations for Plasma-Derived Medicinal Products (PDMPs) in Europe* (Baarn, The Netherlands: Vintura, 2020), 16. This was commissioned by the Plasma Protein Therapeutics Association.
10. Hagen, *Blood Transfusion in Europe*, 188. See also Protein Plasma Therapeutics Association, "What is Plasma?" Available at: www.pptaglobal.org/plasma
11. I discuss this further in Chapter 1.
12. Giuliano Grazzini, Pier Mannuccio, and Fabrizio Oleari, "Plasma Derived Medicinal Products: Demand and Clinical Use," *Blood Transfusion* 11, Suppl. 4 (2013), s1; Plasma Protein Therapeutics Association, "Plasma Protein Therapies," Available at: www.pptaglobal.org/plasma-protein-therapies
13. Hemophilia A and B are hereditary recessive disorders "caused by deficiency or absence of coagulation factors VIII . . . or IX . . . respectively"; its prevalence is roughly 1 in 10000 in the general population. The disease often manifests as bleeding into a joint cavity, with knees, elbows, and ankles most frequently affected. Erik Berntrop and Amy D. Shapiro, "Modern Hemophilia Care," *The Lancet* 379, 9824 (2012), 1447.
14. Von Willebrand Disease is a bleeding disorder which "occurs as a result of decrease in plasma levels or defect in von Willebrand factor which is a large multimeric glycoprotein." It is characterized by a decreased ability of

the blood to clot which leads to "heavy and continuous bleeding after an injury." K. Pavani Bharati and U. Ram Prashanth, "Von Willebrand Disease: An Overview," *Indian Journal of Pharmaceutical Sciences* 73, 1 (2011), 7.

15. Primary immunodeficiency diseases (PIDs) are "a genetically heterogeneous group of disorders that affect distinct components of the innate and adaptive immune system"; there are over 150 such diseases identified with over 120 genes involved. Raif S. Geha et al., "Primary Immunodeficiency Diseases: An Update from the International Union of Immunological Societies Primary Immunodeficiency Diseases Classification Committee," *Journal of Allergy and Clinical Immunology* 120, 4 (2007), 776.

16. Strengers, "Evidence-Based Clinical Indications of Plasma Products and Future Prospects," 3.

17. Evan M. Bloch, et al., "Deployment of Convalescent Plasma for the Prevention and Treatment of COVID-19," *Journal of Clinical Investigation* 130, 6 (2020), 2757–2765; John D. Roback and Jeanette Guarner, "Convalescent Plasma to Treat COVID-19: Possibilities and Challenges," *Journal of the American Medical Association* 323, 16 (2020), 1561–1562.

18. World Health Organization, *World Health Organization Model List of Essential Medicines, 21st List, 2019* (Geneva: World Health Organization, 2019. Licence: CC BY-NC-SA 3.0 IGO), 36.

19. See Paul F.W. Strengers and Harvey G. Klein, "Plasma is a Strategic Resource," *Transfusion* 56, 12 (2016), 3133–3137. I discuss this further in the Conclusion to this volume.

20. For reasons that I will outline in the Conclusion to this volume, my arguments concerning the moral necessity of offering compensation to plasma donors cannot be readily generalized to other bodily products or services, such as whole blood, kidneys, bone marrow, or surrogate pregnancy.

21. Strengers, "Evidence-Based Clinical Indications of Plasma Products and Future Prospects," 5.

22. Cited by Ibid. This data is from 2011.

23. Henry G. Grabowski and Richard L. Manning, "An Economic Analysis of Global Policy Proposals to Prohibit Compensation of Blood Plasma Donors," *International Journal of the Economics of Business* 23, 2 (2016), 155–156.

24. Bloch, et al., "Deployment of Convalescent Plasma for the Prevention and Treatment of COVID-19," 2757–2765; Roback and Guarner, "Convalescent Plasma to Treat COVID-19," 1561–1562.

25. This is a version of the Argument from Force that will be discussed in Chapter 3. That the offers of compensation that are made to prospective donors are too low to be tantalizing is noted in Chapter 5.

26. WHO, *Towards Self-Sufficiency in Safe Blood and Blood Products Based on Voluntary Non-Remunerated Donation* (Geneva: World Health Organization, 2013), 9–10.

27. Grabowski and Manning, "An Economic Analysis of Global Policy Proposals to Prohibit Compensation of Blood Plasma Donors," 151.

28. See Province of Alberta, "Voluntary Blood Donations Act," Assented to (March 30, 2017). Available at: www.qp.alberta.ca/documents/Acts/V05.pdf.

29. See Province of Alberta, "Voluntary Blood Donations Repeal Act," Assented to (December 9, 2020). Available at: www.qp.alberta.ca/Documents/Annual Volumes/2020/ch41_2020.pdf.

30. See Province of British Columbia, "Voluntary Blood Donations Act," Assented to (May 31, 2018). Available at: www.bclaws.ca/civix/document/id/lc/statreg/18030.

31. Bloodwatch, "Securing & Protecting The Canadian Blood Supply Why We Need A Legislative Ban On Paid-Plasma In Canada Senate of Canada & House of Commons Brief," (October 2018), 6.
32. Benjamin E. Hippen, *Organ Sales and Moral Travails: Lessons from the Living Kidney Vendor Program in Iran*, Cato Policy Analysis Series, No. 614 (March 20, 2008).
33. Kieran Healy, *Last Best Gifts: Altruism and the Market for Human Blood and Organs* (Chicago: University of Chicago Press, 2006), 1. The offer of compensation for bone marrow, for example, was only legalized in the United States in 2011. See *Flynn v. Holder*, "United States Court of Appeals for the Ninth Circuit," (December 1, 2011). The exceptions here might be sperm donors and breast milk donors, who, like plasma donors, have a history of receiving compensation for their bodily goods. See, for example, George P. Smith, II, "Through a Test Tube Darkly: Artificial Insemination and the Law," *Michigan Law Review* 67, 1 (1968), 133, and Valerie Fildes, "The English Wet-Nurse and Her Role in Infant Care 1538–1800," *Medical History* 32 (1988), 142–173. Human milk is still a bodily product that is much in demand. See Johanna Kostenzer (on behalf of the EFCNI Working Group on Human Milk Regulation), "Making Human Milk Matter: The Need for EU Regulation," *The Lancet, Child & Adolescent Health* 5, 3 (2021), 161–163.
34. Rose George, for example, describes the potential medical benefits of PDMPs as being such to send "Pharmaceutical Company Finance Departments into a Merry Tailspin of Profit Calculation," *Nine Pints; A Journey Through the Money, Medicine, and Mysteries of Blood* (New York: Metropolitan Books, 2018), 155.
35. I owe this terminology to Iskra Fileva.
36. Julian Koplin, for example, holds that in the absence of any clear evidence concerning the effects of offering compensation on the quantity of kidneys thus produced, it is an open question as to whether or not offering compensation for these organs would increase their supply. "Kidney Sales and Market Regulation: A Reply to Semrau," *The Journal of Medicine and Philosophy* 42, 6 (2017), 661.
37. See Chapter 1. There is one possible exception to this. There has been little work done on the question of whether financially compensating donors for their plasma will attract people away from donating whole blood without compensation to the detriment of its supply – and hence the well-being of patients who need this. However, groundbreaking empirical work on this question by William English and Peter Martin Jaworski shows that this worry is unfounded. They state, "we find no evidence that the introduction of paid plasma has decreased blood donations in Canada. Rather, we find that for every additional 100 plasma collections per city per month, blood clinics have seen a small but significant increase of 8–10 additional blood donations," "The Introduction of Paid Plasma In Canada and the U.S. Has Not Decreased Unpaid Blood Donations," (July 15, 2020), 5. Available at: SSRN: https://ssrn.com/abstract=3653432 or http://dx.doi.org/10.2139/ssrn.3653432
38. See, for example, Taylor, *Stakes and Kidneys*.
39. T.M. Wilkinson, *Ethics and the Acquisition of Organs* (Oxford: Oxford University Press, 2011), 176. Wilkinson noted that Mark J. Cherry, among others, has given "impressively detailed defences of the ethical permissibility of sale" (Ibid., note 24). Wilkinson cites Mark J. Cherry's, *Kidney for Sale By Owner: Human Organs, Transplantation, and the Market* (Washington, DC: Georgetown University Press, 2005).

40. Wilkinson, *Ethics and the Acquisition of Organs*, 176–177.
41. I am tempted to quote A.E. Housman ("What God abandoned, these defended") but this would be inappropriate. In that Epitaph the defense in question was laudable.
42. Here "our" and "their" are merely used to outline how this argument will progress; they do not refer to any particular society.

1 Compensating Plasma Donors Is Safe and Effective

Introduction

I noted in the Introduction to this volume that compensating plasma donors has no adverse effects on patient safety and also leads to more plasma being collected than is secured when compensation is not offered. But these claims are not universally accepted. Appeals to concerns about patient safety and the possible adverse effects that donor compensation might have upon the amount of source plasma that is collected are often made by those who oppose compensated donation. This chapter will put these concerns to rest. This should eliminate any opposition to the compensation of plasma donors that is based on the belief that compensated donation would have adverse effects on patients. With this achieved, any remaining opposition to compensating plasma donors would have to be based on *ethical* objections to this practice.

Shifting the focus of this debate away from the instrumental effects of donor compensation and toward its ethical import is important for two reasons. First, as I outlined in the Introduction, the ethical concerns that putatively support the view that donor compensation is morally impermissible fail to do so. Instead, concerns about donors being rendered vulnerable to, for example, coercion or exploitation will support the view that offering donors compensation is ethically *required* – not that it is ethically impermissible. Second, this ethical focus makes it clear that the prohibition of donor compensation is an example of legal moralism in which the moral views of those with political influence are imposed upon the rest of the population.[1] Given that this approach to legislation is frequently held to be illiberal, its adoption by liberal democracies (such as those EU countries that prohibit donor compensation) stands in need of considerable justification.[2] Shifting the focus of this debate in this way is thus accompanied by a corresponding shift in the burden of proof with this moving from those who support donor compensation to those who defend its prohibition.[3] These two reasons as to why the shift in focus of the debate over donor compensation from the instrumental to the ethical is important are independent of each other. Since this is a work of

DOI: 10.4324/9781003263913-2

moral and not political philosophy, my discussion is sustained by the first of these reasons for this shift and not the second. Having noted this, however, I should also note that an examination of the latter reason is likely to generate further justificatory difficulties for those who support the legal prohibition of donor compensation in a liberal democracy.

Safety and Compensated Plasma Collection

In his exceptionally influential work, *The Gift Relationship* (published in the UK in 1970), Richard M. Titmuss argued that there was *a priori* reason to believe that blood (and blood products) collected from compensated donors would be less safe than that collected from uncompensated donors.[4] Titmuss held that paid donors would treat their blood purely as a market good and its donation as a market transaction.[5] "As a market transaction," writes Titmuss, "information that might have a bearing on the quality of the blood is withheld if possible from the buyer; such information could be detrimental to the price or the sale."[6] This, he claimed, lead to the adoption of deceptive "devices . . . which make it very difficult to screen and exclude as donors drug addicts, alcoholics, and carriers of hepatitis, malaria, and other diseases."[7] Titmuss supported his claims with evidence from 1963 that many "narcotic addicts" who wished to sell blood would "successfully conceal their addiction,"[8] and with an unsubstantiated claim from the 1964 Sixth Annual Meeting of the South Central Association of Blood Banks that "anyone who might need money to buy food or other necessities of life is a person who cannot be trusted."[9]

Before moving to discuss this issue, I should make it clear that despite repeated claims to the contrary all the available evidence definitively establishes that PDMPs manufactured from source plasma obtained from compensated donors are no less safe than those manufactured from source plasma obtained from uncompensated donors. The Government of Canada, for example, notes that "**there have been no confirmed cases of disease transmitted through PDPs in over 2 decades.**"[10] Canadian Blood Services (CBS) similarly categorically states that "drugs made from plasma donated by paid donors are as safe as those made from plasma donated by volunteer donors."[11] This is not merely a Canadian phenomenon. That PDMPs manufactured from source plasma obtained from compensated donors are just as safe as those manufactured from source plasma obtained from uncompensated donors is also recognized by the European Agency for the Evaluation of Medicinal Products, which stated that "[t]here is no evidence from clinical studies and pharmacovigilance that donor remuneration increases the risk of viral transmission via plasma-derived medicinal products, which have been subject to proper screening at donation and a validated viral inactivation/removal step."[12] And in the United States the Plasma Protein Therapeutics

Association – the organization that represents the private-sector manufacturers of plasma protein therapies and the collectors of source plasma used for fractionation – received a backhanded compliment on the safety of the PDMPs manufactured from source plasma from donors compensated by their member companies at the 2011 meeting of the Food and Drug Administration's Blood Products Advisory Committee. At that meeting, Harvey Alter congratulated the private-sector plasma industry and the PPTA for "making the worst blood product imaginable 20 years ago into the safest blood product we have," stating that he thought that the achievement was "a remarkable thing."[13]

Yet despite the acknowledged safety of PDMPs manufactured from source plasma obtained from compensated donors, the view that offering donors compensation will jeopardize patient safety is still influential.[14] In 2013, the WHO published a Global Status Report titled *Towards Self-Sufficiency in Safe Blood and Blood Products based on Voluntary Non-remunerated Donation* in which it held that blood and blood products (including plasma) from compensated donors were less safe than that procured from uncompensated donors.[15] Before I address the WHO's concerns directly I should note that their focus (and hence the focus of those who draw upon the WHO's claims) is misplaced. Since source plasma from compensated donors is exclusively used for the manufacture of PDMPs, the question should not be whether source plasma from compensated donors is as safe as that from uncompensated donors. Instead, the relevant question to ask is the *distinct* question of whether PDMPs that are manufactured from source plasma obtained from compensated donors are as safe as those manufactured from plasma obtained from uncompensated donors. This is the relevant question to ask because it is PDMPs – and not source plasma itself – that are used by patients. And, as I noted earlier, the answer to this question is clearly that they are.

I will now put this issue to one side and address the WHO's (misfocused) question of the relative safety of blood and blood products (including plasma) from compensated and uncompensated donors. But even when focusing on this question the WHO fails to establish that plasma obtained from compensated donors is less safe than that obtained from uncompensated donors.

In support of the claim that blood and blood products (including plasma) from compensated donors is less safe than that procured from uncompensated donors, the WHO noted that in 1997 Bernice Steinhardt testified to the Subcommittee on Human Resources, Committee on Government Reform and Oversight, House of Representatives that commercial plasma donors tested positive for infectious diseases at a greater rate than uncompensated blood donors.[16] The WHO also noted that Volkow et al. found that "in two Mexican-United States border cities, injection drug users hardly donated in Mexico where payment for donations is banned, but they cross-border to the United States where payment is allowed, while denying their risk behavior."[17] The WHO used these observations to support its claim that non-remunerated plasma donors were safer than those that received compensation. This claim was subsequently drawn upon by the Canadian Nurses Association (CNA) in 2014 when they advocated "against initiatives to establish new for-profit plasma collection centres in Canada" on the grounds that plasma procured from compensated donors was less safe than that procured from uncompensated donors.[18] The CNA further supported their position by citing the 1997 Krever Report's view that "Blood and plasma from unpaid donors are safer than blood and plasma from paid donors."[19] The Krever Report was also cited by the Canadian Health Coalition (CHC) in support of their opposition to compensating plasma donors on the grounds that plasma from compensated donors was less safe than that secured from uncompensated donors.[20] More recently, at the January 2017 Executive Board Meeting of the Ontario Public Service Employees Union (OPSEU), it was resolved that "OPSEU call on the Ontario Minister of Health and Premier to demand the Federal government pass similar legislation as the Voluntary Donations Act, and to demand that blood be added to the list of organs that are prohibited from being sold in Canada."[21] This resolution was motivated by Health Canada granting a license to "Exapharma (Canadian Plasma Resources) to open a paid donor [sic] in Saskatchewan, thus endangering the safety of the blood supply for all Canadians."[22]

These concerns with the safety of patients whose treatments are manufactured from source plasma secured from compensated donors are misplaced. But before I move to show why, note that there is something odd about the position of the CNA, the CHC, and the OPSEU: While they all oppose compensating domestic donors of blood and plasma on the grounds that plasma from compensated donors puts patients at risk *none* similarly oppose the importation of PDMPs manufactured from source plasma obtained from foreign donors even though they know that the majority of them are compensated. One possible explanation for this discrepancy is that these organizations believe (falsely) that Canadians are unusually prone to blood-borne diseases. This seems unlikely to be their view. So, another explanation must be offered. Since this book is a work of moral philosophy rather than of empirical political science, I will not pursue this question further here – although I have done elsewhere.[23] I will, however, offer a promissory note that I will pay off in Chapter 6: There is a way to reconcile objecting to offering compensation to prospective domestic plasma donors with allowing the importation of plasma and PDMPs obtained from compensated donors abroad.

The objection to the compensation of domestic donors that is compatible with accepting the importation of plasma and PDMPs obtained from compensated donors abroad clearly cannot be based on claims concerning the dangers of plasma secured from compensated donors. It is thus not an objection that is compatible with the expressed concerns of the CNA, the CHC, and the OPSEU. To return to the immediate issue at hand I will now address their (putative) concerns about the practical effects of donor compensation on the supply of blood and blood products.[24]

To see why these concerns are misplaced consider the sources cited by the WHO. Steinhardt's 1997 testimony led to a significant increase in the regulatory oversight to which the plasma fractionation industry was subject.[25] As a result of this, it was noted in a 1998 Report that while "paid plasma donors are over one and a half times more likely to donate potentially infectious units," "a number of recent initiatives by the source plasma industry greatly reduce the chances of these units being pooled for manufacturing."[26] This report was provided to the same Subcommittee to which Steinhardt testified but was not acknowledged by the WHO in its 2013 Report. The WHO also ignored the fact that Steinhardt's testimony was delivered 24 years ago, prior to the current use of modern screening techniques for viruses. The introduction of Nucleic Acid Amplification Technology (NAT) testing, for example, allows for screening of the non-lipid enveloped viruses such as HBV hepatitis B virus (HBV), hepatitis C virus (HCV), and HIV.[27] These viruses were specifically identified in the 1998 Report as being those whose transmission by PDMPs was of concern.[28] Thus, while Steinhardt's testimony was rightly influential in reforming the plasma industry the data that she cited was peculiar to the time and place of her testimony. It thus has no evidential relevance to the current discussion of the safety of plasma procured from compensated donors.

Just as the WHO did not address data relevant to the question of the safety of compensated donation that was produced subsequently to Steinhardt's 1997 testimony so too did it fail to acknowledge relevant information that had been provided in response to the work of Volkow et al. But before turning to consider this note that the WHO's account of the work of Volkow et al. might give the impression that significant numbers of injection drug users (IDU) were crossing the US–Mexico border to donate their plasma for compensation. But Volkow et al. are clear that the cohort of IDUs that they studied were receiving compensation for their plasma a median of 13 years *prior* to their 2005 survey with only three donors receiving compensation in the period 2003–2005.[29] Moreover, as Penrod et al. note in response to Volkow et al., it can be deduced that the majority of the IDUs that they surveyed attempted to donate plasma prior to the 1980s since they specified "manual plasmapheresis as the collection technology."[30] This procedure has been "superseded by automated plasmapheresis for over 20 years."[31] Penrod et al. (rightly) concede that it is worrying that "two" IDUs donated plasma.[32] But they go on to note that the safety of PDMPs would not be compromised even if the attempted "exclusion of high-risk individuals through donor selection" failed to identify a donor who was an IDU. This is because two other sets of procedures are in place to ensure patient safety: "the testing of all plasma for relevant pathogens" and "the elimination of pathogens through manufacture."[33] And, again, it is the safety of the PDMPs that is at issue – not that of the source plasma.

The procedures involved in the "exclusion of high-risk individuals through donor selection" that Penrod et al. mention are exceptionally rigorous. Under the plasma industry's voluntary International Quality Plasma Program (IQPP), potential donors of source plasma are divided into "Applicant Donors" and "Qualified Donors."[34] An "Applicant Donor" is a prospective donor who has not qualified as a "Qualified Donor" within the previous six months prior to presenting to donate. To become a "Qualified Donor," a person must undergo a physical examination by an appropriate healthcare professional and be checked against the National Donor Deferral Registry (NDDR). (The NDDR contains "the names of individuals who have previously tested positive for HIV, HBV, or HCV at plasma collection centers.")[35] In jurisdictions where checking the NDDR is "not applicable by law," an Applicant Donor must be checked against the plasma company's donor management system.[36] If a state or federal donor deferral registry also exists, then the Applicant Donor must be checked against this as well. The prospective donor must also be educated so that she understands the processes that she is consenting to and the risks involved. Once these steps have been successfully completed, the Applicant Donor must donate a complete (sample) unit of plasma and successfully pass "donor screening and testing non-reactive for HIV, HBV and HCV based on all applicable regulatory and IQPP requirements."[37] However, while the donor's testing negative for a known virus at the time of her initial donation is necessary for the plasma she donates to be used in the manufacture of PDMPs it is not sufficient for this. For her donated plasma to be used in the manufacture of PDMPs, the donor must return again to donate within six months of her initial donation. She then undergoes the same rigorous screening procedures as before. If she is again negative after this inventory hold period, then she will become a Qualified Donor and her plasma can be used.[38] This means that plasma procured from a one-time donor is not used in the manufacture of PDMPs.[39] No units of plasma are accepted from an Applicant Donor until she has become a Qualified Donor, and if a Qualified Donor does not return to donate within six months from qualifying, she will be reclassified as an Applicant Donor.[40]

Further safety precautions are taken once source plasma enters the manufacturing process.[41] The "gold standard" for the viral inactivation of plasma products consists of two stages. The first stage "is designed to inactivate most enveloped viruses, including HIV, HBV, and HCV, and usually involves the use of solvent detergents."[42] This procedure is then followed by heat treatment processes that are designed to inactivate both enveloped and non-enveloped viruses.[43] In addition to these two processes, nanofiltration is used to further reduce the risk of transmission of non-enveloped viruses.[44] Nucleic acid amplification technology (NAT) testing is also used "to reduce the potential for 'window period' plasma donations to enter the manufacturing pool" through the detection of viral DNA.[45] (A "window period" refers to the time period between a person's being infected with a virus such as HIV or HCV and the time when she has begun to produce antibodies that can be detected through conventional testing.)[46] So successful have these (and earlier) safety procedures been that there has been no transmission of HIV or HBV through a US-licensed plasma derivative since 1987.[47] There has been no transmission of HCV through a US-licensed plasma derivative since 1994 – and that occurred only once as a design flaw in a manufacturing plant.[48]

Since these safety procedures apply to plasma procured from both compensated and uncompensated donors, there is no difference between the safety of PDMPs produced from source plasma secured from compensated donors and that of those that are produced from source plasma secured from uncompensated donors. As I noted earlier, it has been expressly acknowledged by multiple government agencies across the world that the safety of PDMPs produced from source plasma obtained from compensated donors is the same as that of those made from source plasma secured from uncompensated donors. The Government of Canada, for example, states in its "Backgrounder Paper – Plasma Donations in Canada" that "[t]he plasma collected from paid and unpaid donors is equally safe, because every donor is treated the same."[49] This is not surprising. The safety of a PDMP depends not on whether the Qualified Donors whose plasma went into its manufacturing received cash as they left the center in which they donated but on their being qualified donors whose donated plasma was then processed according to the "gold standard" of PDMP manufacturing.

Unfortunately, this is not acknowledged either by the WHO or by those (such as the CAN, CHC, and OPSEU) who also assert that compensated donation would put patient safety at risk.[50] This lack of acknowledgment of the safety of PDMPs manufactured from source plasma from compensated donors is likely to be the result of three factors.

First, as I noted earlier, the authors of the WHO Report have ignored the crucial fact that source plasma, unlike whole blood, is not infused directly into patients but is extensively processed during the manufacturing of PDMPs.[51] This oversight would explain why they cited Volkow et al.'s identification of plasma donation by three IUDs as evidence that the use of plasma from compensated donors is unsafe for patients. This proper concern with patient safety should have been allayed by the recognition both that under current IQPP requirements these donors would not have become Qualified Donors and that even if they had become Qualified, the safety precautions in place during the manufacturing process would have detected or inactivated any viral load present.[52] Given this, it is not surprising that as long ago as 1997 (i.e., before the introduction of many current manufacturing processes and IQPP requirements) John Keown – a *critic* of compensated donation – acknowledged that

> [p]lasma products which are derived from paid and well-screened donors and which are subjected to effective viral inactivation procedures are likely to be much safer than plasma from unpaid and poorly-screened donors which is not virally inactivated. In other words, non-payment no more ensures safety than payment precludes safety.[53]

The view that PDMPs manufactured from source plasma collected from compensated donors is less safe than those manufactured from source plasma collected from uncompensated donors is merely a "moribund myth."[54]

Second, views on the safety of products produced from source plasma secured from compensated donors might still be influenced by the long shadow of the less robust collection and processing practices of the 1960s, 1970s, and 1980s that led to the introduction of both HCV and then HIV into many countries' supply of blood and blood products.[55] During this period, contaminated blood and plasma were secured from both compensated and uncompensated donors.[56] However, that contaminated blood and plasma were secured from uncompensated donors as well as compensated donors was (and is) often overlooked. This is likely because many commentators were (and are) influenced by Richard Titmuss' argument that while donors with pro-social motivations would refrain from donating if they believed that this would put others at risk, donors motivated by financial (i.e., selfish) considerations would be motivated to lie about their health status so they could donate and be compensated.[57] The blame for the public health crises involving blood was thus placed firmly (if unfairly) on the shoulders of the commercial sector.

Finally, independently of whether such blame is justified this has no bearing on the current safety of PDMPs manufactured from source plasma procured from compensated donors. Advances in biotechnology and revisions in the regulatory environment have led to dramatic changes in both the collection of source plasma and the manufacturing of PDMPs that together ensure that current practices are vastly improved from those of the 1970s and 1980s.[58] To hold that PDMPs manufactured from the plasma of compensated donors that was procured and processed under current practices are unsafe on the grounds that blood and blood products procured from compensated donors generations before were unsafe is utterly absurd. It is the bioethical equivalent of someone claiming that a 2015 Ford Fusion is unsafe on the basis of believing that a 1980 Ford Pinto was a "death trap" as it risked exploding when it was rear-ended.[59]

The Effectiveness of Compensated Plasma Collection

Just as it is not universally accepted that PDMPs manufactured from plasma secured from compensated donors pose no additional risk to patient safety above that imposed by PDMPs manufactured from source plasma procured from uncompensated donors so, too, it is not universally accepted that compensating donors will lead to an increase in the supply of plasma.[60]

Before moving to discuss this issue, I should again emphasize that despite repeated claims to the contrary all the available evidence shows clearly that offering compensation to prospective plasma donors will increase the amount of plasma that is available for manufacture into PDMPs. (As with my earlier discussion of safety, then, the following discussion is intended both to charitably outline why some persons continue to believe that offers of compensation have no positive effect on the amount of plasma collected and to demonstrate that this belief is false.) Much of the plasma obtained in the United States is obtained from compensated donors. In 2017, the United States supplied 71% of all source plasma globally and 65% of world plasma for fractionation.[61] This data clearly establishes that rather than diminishing the world's supply of plasma that is made available for eventual patient use the offer of compensation is critical to securing it.[62] I will present further evidence for this claim in the following. My immediate purpose here – as with my introduction to my discussion of the safety issues associated with the question of donor compensation, mentioned earlier – is to make it clear from the outset that despite the contrary beliefs of some it should be uncontroversial that donor compensation is necessary to obtain sufficient source plasma to meet medical need.

I will now turn to outline the contrary view and show why it is mistaken.

Standard economic theory holds that offering compensation for a good or service that was previously procured from uncompensated donors would increase its supply. However, there is evidence that shows that this is not always the case. Indeed, as Erik Malmqvist has noted, "[s]ome opponents of markets in body parts even think that payment may *decrease* the number [or amount] . . . available by discouraging those who would otherwise donate for free."[63] It is the views of such people that I address in this section.

The explanation of why the number or amount of body parts procured after compensation for them is offered begins by distinguishing between two types of preferences. The first type consists of the preferences that an individual has for securing material payoffs for herself. The second type consists of her "social preferences." These are her preferences to act on such motives as "altruism, reciprocity, intrinsic pleasure in helping others, inequity aversion, ethical commitments, and other motives that induce people to help others more than would an own-material-payoff maximizing individual."[64] The degree to which a person's social preferences motivate her to perform a certain action (e.g., donate plasma) could either be enhanced by the provision of incentives that appeal to her preferences to secure material payoffs for herself or be reduced by this.[65] If an offer of incentives to perform an action that appeal to preferences to secure material payoffs for herself *reduces* her social preference for performing that action, then this might diminish her overall motivation to do it. If this occurs widely then the offer of incentives would decrease the occurrence of the actions whose performance they were intended to stimulate. Moreover, not only might the offer of incentives be counterproductive, it might be *irrevocably* counterproductive. The offer of an incentive to perform an action that persons previously performed to satisfy their social preferences might lead them to a different understanding of the action in question. Uncompensated plasma donors, for example, might initially understand their donation as being a "priceless gift of life" and be motivated to donate by a social preference to aid others. The introduction of an incentive to donate could change this understanding of the act of donation so that it is no longer considered to be a "priceless gift" but the sale of a good with a particular economic value. If the psychological benefits that donors received from giving this "priceless gift" were more valuable to them than the material benefits that they were offered, and if the material benefits were too low to motivate them to donate, then the offer of compensation would reduce, not increase, the amount of plasma that is procured.[66] This revised understanding of plasma donation might be retained even if compensation is no longer offered. If this were so, then former plasma donors who were motivated to donate the "priceless gift of life" would not go back to donating once compensation was removed. They would now understand their donation to be merely an economic transaction – and one whose material benefit to them has now moved from being low to nonexistent.[67]

This account of how incentives could lead to a reduction (perhaps even an *irrevocable* reduction) in the performance of actions that they are intended to stimulate has empirical support. In one of the best-known studies of this phenomenon, Uri Gneezy and Aldo Rustichini examined the effect that the imposition of a monetary fine had on the behavior of parents who were late in picking up their children from an Israeli day care center. They found that once the fine was introduced there was a significant increase in the number of parents who were late in picking up their children. They also found that there was no reduction in the number of late parents once the fine was removed.[68] Similar results have been found by Irlenbusch and Sliwka who investigated a simple principal-agent problem in which a principal sets a wage and then an agent chooses an effort level in response with the payoff for the principal being fixed by the effort of the agent. They found that in the second setting when the principal could offer a fixed wage and a piece rate to supplement it, agents produced less effort than when they were only offered a fixed wage. When the same treatment was then switched to one where only fixed rates could be paid, agents' efforts declined further.[69] Other studies that did not study the longer term effects on persons' motivation to perform the action that the incentive was intended to elicit have confirmed that in a range of settings the offer of certain incentives decreases rather than increases the desired behavior.[70]

Since donors who provide plasma in legal regimes where financial compensation is prohibited are (it is assumed) motivated to donate by their social preferences it is possible that the introduction of financial compensation for donation could result in some of them either ceasing to donate or donating with less frequency. If these donors' decrease in donation levels is not offset by an increase in donations from new (qualified) donors who are primarily motivated to donate to secure materials payoffs for themselves then the introduction of compensation will lead to a decrease in the overall amount of plasma that is collected.[71] The question of what effect the offer of compensation would have on the supply of plasma is an empirical one. As such, it can only be settled by appeal to data. As J.D. Jasper et al. noted, "[n]othing short of a market test can demonstrate conclusively the impact that incentives would have on . . . supply."[72] Fortunately – and unlike in many other debates over the ethics of compensating the donors of body parts – such a "market test" is available in the case of plasma.[73]

And this test conclusively demonstrates not only that donor compensation does not lead to a reduction in the amount of plasma collected but that it leads to significant increases. In Europe and Scandinavia, the countries with the highest rates of plasma collected for fractionation are Germany and the Czech Republic, both of whom allow compensation to be offered to donors. In 2011, the Czech Republic collected 48.98 L of plasma for fractionation per 1000 inhabitants; Germany collected 36.75 L per 1000 inhabitants.[74] By comparison, the rates of plasma collection for fractionation in countries that do not allow compensation to be offered to donors were significantly lower.[75] In 2011, the highest rates of plasma for fractionations secured by countries that did not allow donor compensation was found in The Netherlands (19.9 L per 1000 inhabitants), Belgium (16.56 L per 1000 inhabitants), and Sweden (14.42 L).[76] By contrast, in 2012, the United States (which allows donor compensation) secured 75.31 L per 1000 inhabitants.[77]

I must acknowledge that the ability of plasma centers to offer compensation to their donors is not the only reason why the United States is able to collect so much plasma in comparison to European countries. Restrictions on donor frequency and volume are more stringent in Europe than in the United States. The United States allows 104 donations per donor a year with a maximum of two donations a week while the Council of

Europe allows 33 donations per donor per year with a maximum of once a week.[78] The United States has set 800 mL as the maximum volume of plasma that can be collected per donation while the Council of Europe permits 750 mL.[79] (Both of these figures are dependent on the weight of the donor.)[80] The United States allows a maximum volume of 83 L of plasma to be donated per donor per year while the Council of Europe permits 25 L per year.[81] However, the effects of the more rational regulations in the United States on the volume of plasma that it collects should not be overstated. In 2012, George Brooks Schreiber and Mary Clare Kimber collected demographic and donation data for c. 1.5 million donors who in 2012 provided c. 25.2 million donations from seven participating plasma procurement agencies in the United States.[82] They found that the average number of donations per donor (in 2012) was 17.5. They also found that 49% of donors donated less than or equal to 10 donations a year, and 14% made over 50 donations a year. Only 0.3% of donors donated more than 100 times a year. Moreover, only 62% of donors donated the maximum volume of plasma allowed.[83] Taken together with the data from Germany and the Czech Republic, this demonstrates that it is not the more rational regulations of the United States that enables it to be the world's largest securer of source plasma. It is the fact that it allows plasma centers to offer compensation to their donors.

The concern that offering compensation to donors would reduce the amount of plasma collected is thus unfounded. But despite the frequent appeal to the possibility of motivational crowding by those who hold that offering donors compensation could lower the amount of plasma that is collected, the fact that offering donors compensation increases the amount of plasma collected will come as no surprise to anyone familiar with the relevant academic literature. As the title of a widely cited paper by Uri Gneezy and Aldo Rustichini indicates ("Pay enough – or don't pay at all") while it is possible that offering a small incentive to persons to encourage them to perform a desired action might result in fewer instances of that action, a larger incentive could overcome this motivational crowding and result in the desired outcome.[84] The success of the United States, Germany, and the Czech Republic in securing source plasma clearly indicates that the level of compensation that they are offering is "enough" to overcome any possible motivational crowding that might have occurred.

Plasma Donation and Donor Health

Before moving to conclude this chapter, I should address a concern that might be raised concerning the ability of donors in the United States to donate more than their European counterparts: That increased donation might have an adverse effect on donor health.[85]

While the donation of plasma is a "very safe procedure," there is concern that it is accompanied by risks to donor health, including increased iron deficiency and reduction in immunoglobulin levels.[86] Concerns have also been expressed about the hypothetical possibility of an increased risk of "arteriosclerotic cardiovascular disease due to plasmapheresis-induced chronic plasma protein loss," and the possibility that donors' serum protein levels could decrease.[87]

Since source plasma donors have red blood cells returned during apheresis, the risk of plasma donation leading to iron deficiency would seem to be low. And this is indeed the case. As George B. Schreiber et al. have shown even frequent source plasma donation does not adversely affect iron stores, a finding that substantiates the view that "circulating plasma iron represents a small portion of total body iron."[88]

The other concerns about donor health mentioned earlier have also been allayed. In 1993, Michael B. Rodell reported the results of a retrospective study in which the records of plasma donors who had been donating for ten or more years were reviewed. Rodell reported that this study showed that there were no significant differences with respect to the mean values of donor's body weight, microhematocrit, total protein, and individual serum proteins between donors who donated < 12 times a year, 12–24 times a year, 25–48 times a year, and > 48 times a year.[89] This survey did not, however, include information about donors who had ceased to donate. It was thus possible that the data failed to reflect any adverse effects of donation that had been experienced by donors and which had led them to discontinue donating. To determine if donors ceased donating for health-related reasons Michael B. Rodell and M.L. Lee conducted a survey to determine why donors ceased donating. They focused on "[d]onors who had successfully undergone plasmapheresis at least 20 times within a recent 6-month period but who had failed to appear for at least 30 days subsequent to their last donation."[90] They found that the primary reasons that donors stated for ceasing to donate were socioeconomic rather than health-related; they stated that they ceased donating as the remuneration was no longer needed, they faced increased time constraints, had relocated, or their work schedules precluded donation.[91]

Similar effects were found in a later study conducted in Germany by S. Bechtloff et al.[92] Bechtloff et al. observed 72 donors over the course of a three-year period who were moved from a moderate plasmapheresis program to an intensive one.[93] (The initial moderate program was one in which donors had "donated between 35 and 38 plasma units [650 ml plus citrate anticoagulant] within the year prior to inclusion.")[94] In the more intensive program to which donors agreed to be moved the maximum number of donations was 60 a year. Donors who weighed < 70 kg (c. 154 lb) were asked to donate 750 mL of plasma (including citrate) each session, at least once a week over 36 months. Donors who weighed

≥ 70 kg were able to volunteer to donate 850 mL of plasma (including citrate) each session, at least once a week over 36 months.[95] Bechtloff et al. note that their more intensive program of plasma donation led to the number of donations in their study group being "much higher than the US average of 15–17 sessions per year."[96] As such, they note, "the programme of plasmapheresis undergone by our donors was an intensive one when compared internationally."[97] Bechtloff et al. monitored each donor's total serum protein (TSP), albumin, and immunoglobulin G (IgG) levels regularly throughout the study.[98] They also monitored their parameters of red cell and iron metabolism and their cardiovascular risk factors.[99] They noted that the percentage of subjects with "TSP, and/or IgG values below threshold levels, or exhibiting iron store depletion (as indicated by ferritin levels below 12 ng/ml), did not increase significantly during observation."[100] They also noted that "[m]arkers of increased cardiovascular risk neither differed significantly between donors and non-donor controls at baseline, nor changed significantly during observation."[101] They concluded that these results indicate that "long-term intensive donor plasmapheresis did not compromise the individuals' suitability to donate plasma" on health grounds.[102] This is not surprising. As Schulzki et al. have observed, "[l]ong-term intensive donor plasmapheresis programmes have been carried out in the USA for decades without serious clinical complications."[103]

Conclusion

Offering financial compensation to plasma donors neither compromises the safety of patients nor leads to a reduction in the amount of plasma collected. Nor does it motivate donors to behave in ways that compromise their health. Indeed, offering a sufficient (i.e., nontrivial) amount of compensation to prospective plasma donors will significantly increase the amount of source plasma that is collected. Since collecting less plasma will make PDMPs less accessible to patients, the onus is on the defenders of prohibition to provide an argument that is robust enough to justify jeopardizing the health of patients in this way. If no such arguments are forthcoming, then patients will have been harmed for no apparent reason. And this is clearly wrongful.

But this is not the only way in which the objection that donor compensation will deter some donors from donating backfires on the defenders of prohibition. That low levels of compensation will crowd out some donors from donating can be explained by holding that the level of compensation will communicate to some donors that their donations are not as valuable as they thought that they were when compensation was not offered. When provided with this information, some donors will cease donating as they have come to believe that the (low) value of their donation is outweighed by their opportunity costs. For some donors, then, the information that compensation can convey concerning the value of their donation will be relevant for their decision as to whether or not they should donate. Since this is so (as I will argue in the next chapter), prohibiting donor compensation will preclude some donors from giving their informed consent to donate. Donor compensation is thus required not only out of concern for the health of patients. It is also required out of concern for the autonomy and well-being of donors.

Notes

1. Although offering compensation to plasma donors is widely prohibited in Canada, there is evidence that the Canadian public overwhelmingly supports donor compensation. See Nicola Lacetera and Mario Macis, "Moral Nimby-Ism? Understanding Societal Support for Monetary Compensation to Plasma Donors in Canada," *Law and Contemporary Problems* 81 (2018), 83–105.
2. That this approach to legislation is illiberal is noted by, for example, John Stuart Mill, *On Liberty* (Indianapolis: Hackett Publishing Co., 1978), and David O. Brink, "Retributivism and Legal Moralism," *Ratio Juris* 25, 4 (2012), 496.
3. Note that the immediate burden here is to justify legal moralism not to justify the prohibition of donor compensation. The latter issue can only be addressed once the legal moralists who would prohibit donor compensation on moral grounds have justified their approach. The burden of proof thus lies within the realm of political, not moral, philosophy. For a discussion of burden of proof arguments in bioethics, see Janet Radcliffe Richards, *The Ethics of Transplants: Why Careless Thought Costs Lives* (Oxford: Oxford University Press, 2012), and "Not a Defence of Organ Markets," *Journal of Practical Ethics* 7, 3 (2019), 56–58, and Julian J. Koplin and Michael J. Selgelid, "The Burden of Proof in Bioethics," *Bioethics* 29, 9 (2015), 597–603, and "Kidney Sales and the Burden of Proof," *Journal of Practical Ethics* 7, 3 (2019), 32–53.
4. Richard M. Titmuss, *The Gift Relationship: From Human Blood to Social Policy* (New York: Vintage Books, 1971), Chapter 5.
5. In addition to the "paid donor," Titmuss identified three other types of donors who would be motivated to provide blood or blood products to receive compensation, and so to whom these concerns would also apply. These are the "professional donor" (who yield blood for payment, but who do so on a more regular basis than paid donors), the "paid-induced voluntary donor" (who expects to be paid for his donation, but who claims not to be primarily motivated by payment), and the "captive voluntary donor" (who donates as a result of a complex mix of social pressures, some of which might include financial reward). Titmuss, *The Gift Relationship*, 77–88.
6. Ibid., 76. It will be argued in the next chapter that the moral concern with the withholding of relevant information should lead one to object to the prohibition of donor compensation.
7. Ibid. The medical and regulatory environment that Titmuss was writing (in the 1960s) was very different from that which exists today.
8. Robert F. Norris, H. Phelps Potter, Jr., and John G. Reinhold, "Present Status of Hepatic Function Tests in the Detection of Carriers of Viral Hepatitis," *Transfusion* 3, 3 (1963), 208. Cited by Titmuss, *The Gift Relationship*, 76, note 4.

9. F. Del Prete, "A Study of the IP Factor in Blood Donors," *Presented at the Sixth Annual Meeting of the South Central Association of Blood Banks, Oklahoma City* (March 1964), 5. Cited by Titmuss, *The Gift Relationship*, 76.

10. Bold text in original. Health Canada, *Protecting Access to Immune Globulins for Canadians. Final report of the Expert Panel on the Immune Globulin Product Supply and Related Impacts in Canada* (Ottawa: Health Canada, 2018), 8.

11. Canadian Blood Services, "Our Commitment to Increasing Plasma Sufficiency in Canada," Available at: www.blood.ca/en/about-us/media/plasma/plasma-sufficiency

12. European Agency for the Evaluation of Medicinal Products, "CPMP Position Statement Non-Remunerated and Remunerated Donors: Safety and Supply of Plasma-Derived Medicinal Products," (May 30, 2002), 2.

13. Food and Drug Administration Center for Biologics Evaluation and Research, "Blood Products Advisory Committee Meeting, Transcript Prepared by CASET Associates Ltd," (April 28, 2011). Harvey Alter was a member of the Department of Transfusion Medicine at the National Institutes of Health. His remark occurs on p. 38 of the transcript.

14. Alastair V. Campbell, Cecilia Tan, and F. Elias Boujaoude, for example, claim that blood (and by implication blood products, such as plasma) is safest when secured from unpaid donations. Alastair V. Campbell, Cecilia Tan, and F. Elias Boujaoude, "The Ethics of Blood Donation: Does Altruism Suffice?" *Biologicals* 40, 3 (2012), 171. In support of this claim, they cite Titmuss', *The Gift Relationship* and the World Health Organisation, "Blood Safety and Availability," Available at: www.who.int/mediacentre/factsheets/fs279/en/index.html. As I will note in the following, Titmuss was writing about the procurement of blood and blood products in the 1950s and 1960s and so his claims concerning the relative safety of blood and blood products from compensated and uncompensated donors are out of date and thus irrelevant to the current debate. Note, too, that claims about the relative safety of blood from compensated and uncompensated donors will not support similar claims concerning the relative safety of source plasma from compensated and uncompensated since (as I will discuss in the Conclusion to this volume) source plasma is not transfused but used to manufacture PDMPs. Moreover, as Kieran Healy has documented, the relative safety of blood from compensated and uncompensated donors is contingent upon the degree to which blood-borne diseases are correlated with the populations from which these classes of donors are drawn. It is possible that the association of disease with uncompensated donors and health with compensated donors will be "turned upside down" if a pathogen becomes prevalent in the former population but not the latter (as happened with HIV). See Healy, *Last Best Gifts*, 92.

15. WHO, *Towards Self-Sufficiency in Safe Blood and Blood Products*.

16. Ibid., 10. The WHO cites Bernice Steinhardt, *Enhancing Safeguards Would Strengthen the Nation's Blood Supply* (United States General Accounting Office, June 5, 1997), 5–6. Available at: https://www.gao.gov/assets/t-hehs-97-143.pdf

17. WHO, *Towards Self-Sufficiency in Safe Blood and Blood Products*, 10. The WHO cites P. Volkow et al., "Cross-Border Paid Plasma Donation Among Injection Drug Users in Two Mexico – U.S. Border Cities," *International Journal of Drug Policy* 20, 5 (2009), 409–412.

18. Canadian Nurses Association, "Resolution 4: Protect Canada's Blood Supply by Rejecting For-Profit Plasma Collection," Available at: https://rnao.

ca/sites/rnao-ca/files/Resolution_4_-_Protect_Canadas_Blood_Supply_by_Rejecting_for-Profit_Plasma_Collection.pdf

19. Ibid., 1. The Canadian Nurses Association cites Horace Krever, *The Commission of Inquiry on the Blood System in Canada – Final Report* (Ottawa, Ontario: Publications du ministère de la Santé et des Services Sociaux, 1997), 1048.

20. Canadian Health Coalition, "Unpaid Plasma and Blood Donation," Available at: www.healthcoalition.ca/unpaid-plasma-and-blood-donations/

21. OPSEU, "Minutes of the January 25–26 Executive Board Meeting," Available at: https://opseu.org/information/minutes/minutes-of-the-january-25-26-2017-executive-board-meeting/16160/

22. Ibid. As its name suggests, Canadian Plasma Resources only collects source plasma and not whole blood; the OPSEU's concern should thus be with the safety of Canada's plasma supply, not its whole blood supply.

23. See James Stacey Taylor, "The Ethics and Politics of Blood Plasma Donation: The Case in Canada," *International Journal of Applied Philosophy* 34, 1 (2020), 89–103.

24. Why these concerns might be merely putative than real is explained in Ibid.

25. Michael A. Friedman, "Testimony on the GAO Report on 'Blood Plasma Safety.'" (September 9, 1998). Available at: www.hhs.gov/asl/testify/t980909a.html

26. United States General Accounting Office, "Plasma Product Risks are Low if Good Manufacturing Practices Are Followed," *Report to the Chairman, Subcommittee on Human Resources, Committee on Government Reform and Oversight, House of Representatives* (September 9, 1998), 2. Available at: www.gao.gov/assets/hehs-98-205.pdf (Accessed March 29, 2021).

27. Anne-Maree Farrell, *The Politics of Blood: Ethics, Innovation, and the Regulation of Risk* (Cambridge: Cambridge University Press, 2012), 115. Enveloped viruses are viruses whose membranes contain lipid molecules. Ibid., note 79.

28. United States General Accounting Office. "Plasma Product Risks are Low," 1.

29. Volkow et al., "Cross-Border Paid Plasma Donation," 409.

30. J. Penrod et al. "Response to Volkow P et al. – Cross-Border Paid Plasma Donation Among Injection Drug Users in Two Mexico – U.S. Border Cities – International Journal of Drug Policy 20 (2009) 409–412," *International Journal of Drug Policy* 21 (2010), 343.

31. Ibid.

32. Ibid. They are in error to state that the number was two; it was three. See Volkow et al., "Cross-Border Paid Plasma Donation," 409. This does not affect the argument of Penrod et al.

33. Penrod et al., "Response to Volkow P et al.," 343.

34. Protein Plasma Therapeutics Association, "IQPP Qualified Donor Standard Version 4.0," (June 25, 2014). Available at: www.pptaglobal.org/images/IQPP/QualifiedDonorStdFinal1.pdf

35. Farrell, *The Politics of Blood*, 114.

36. Protein Plasma Therapeutics Association, "IQPP Qualified Donor Standard Version 4.0."

37. Ibid.

38. Farrell, *The Politics of Blood*, 114.

39. Ibid. Farrell cites V. Grifols, "Financing Plasma Proteins: Unique Challenges," *Pharmaceutical Policy and Law* 7 (2006), 189. Note that this is the case for fractionators using IQPP-certified plasma. I thank Joshua Penrod for clarifying this for me.

40. Protein Plasma Therapeutics Association, "IQPP Qualified Donor Standard Version 4.0."
41. For a technical overview of these processes, see Thierry Burnouf, "An Overview of Plasma Fractionation," *Annals of Blood* 3, 33 (2018), 1–10.
42. Farrell, *The Politics of Blood*, 115.
43. Ibid. A non-enveloped virus is a virus that contains mainly proteins. Ibid., n. 79.
44. Ibid.
45. Ibid.
46. Ibid.
47. E. Tabor, "The Epidemiology of Virus Transmission by Plasma Derivatives: Clinical Studies Verifying the Lack of Transmission of Hepatitis B and C Viruses and HIV Type 1," *Transfusion* 39 (1999), 1166.
48. Ibid., 1160.
49. Government of Canada, "Backgrounder Paper – Plasma Donations in Canada," Available at: www.canada.ca/en/health-canada/services/drugs-health-products/public-involvement-consultations/biologics-radiopharma ceuticals-genetic-therapies/backgrounder-paper-plasma-donations-canada. html
50. Or, perhaps, *claim* to believe – see note 21.
51. Healy, *Last Best Gifts*, 75.
52. One might be skeptical that the WHO overlooked in this way the different uses to which whole blood and source plasma are put. But the 2013 Report is riddled with error, including the citation of sources to support a point when the source supports the opposite point, portmanteau citations (i.e., where the source cited does not exist, but instead is an amalgam of two different sources), and failures to cite literature that corrected its cited sources. See James Stacey Taylor, "A Scandal in Geneva: Culpable Negligence and the WHO's 2013 Report on National Self-Sufficiency in Blood and Blood Products," *International Journal of Applied Philosophy* 28, 2 (2014), 219–234, See also my "WTF WHO?" *HEC Forum* 27 (2015), 287–300.
53. John Keown, "The Gift of Blood in Europe: An Ethical Defence of EC Directive 89/381," *Journal of Medical Ethics* 23 (1997), 96–100.
54. J-P. Allain, "Volunteer Safer Than Replacement Donor Blood: A Myth Revealed by Evidence," *ISBT Science Series* 5, 1 (2010), 169. Allain was here referring to blood but the point stands with respect to PDMPs also.
55. Krever, *Final Report*, 18.
56. Ibid., 132, 227. See also Healy, *Last Best Gifts*, 91–109.
57. Titmuss, *The Gift Relationship*, 76. This argument was repeated by Krever, *Final Report*, 1047.
58. Thierry Burnouf, "Modern Plasma Fractionation," *Transfusion Medicine Reviews* 21, 2 (2007), 101–117.
59. The 2015 Ford Fusion earned a five-star safety rating from United States Government National Highway Traffic Safety Administration (see: www. nhtsa.gov/vehicle/2015/FORD/FUSION/4%252520DR/FWD). For the original account of the dangers of the Pinto, see Mark Dowie, "Pinto Madness," *Mother Jones* (September/October 1977). Available at: www.mother jones.com/politics/1977/09/pinto-madness/. The public perception of the Ford Pinto, however, appears not to fit with the facts; see Gary T. Schwartz, "The Myth of the Ford Pinto Case," *Rutgers Law Review* 43 (1991), 1013–1068.
60. WHO, *Towards Self-Sufficiency in Safe Blood and Blood Products*, 5.
61. Prevot and Jolles, "Global Immunoglobulin Supply," 560.

62. This point would be even more starkly made by citing data presented by J. Mercier Ythier, who claimed that in 2014 the United States provided more than 70% of the world's demand for plasma, with 95% of this being obtained from compensated donors. See J. Mercier Ythier, "The Contested Market of Plasma," *Transfusion Clinique et Biologique* 27, 1 (2020), 54. Unfortunately, Ythier does not cite a source for his claim that 95% of plasma secured in the United States that year was from compensated donors.

63. Erik Malmqvist, "Are Bans on Kidney Sales Unjustifiably Paternalistic?" *Bioethics* 28, 3 (2014), 111. See Koplin, "Kidney Sales and Market Regulation: A Reply to Semrau," 661.

64. This distinction is taken from Samuel Bowles and Sandra Polanía-Reyes, "Economic Incentives and Social Preferences: Substitutes or Complements?" *Journal of Economic Literature* 50, 2 (2012), 370

65. Ibid., 371.

66. These issues are discussed further in Chapters 6 and 7.

67. The importance of this for the ability of donors to give their informed consent is discussed in Chapter 2.

68. Uri Gneezy and Aldo Rustichini, "A Fine Is a Price," *Journal of Legal Studies* 29, 1 (2000), 1–17.

69. Bernd Irlenbusch and Dirk Sliwka, *Incentives, Decision Frames, and Motivation Crowding Out – An Experimental Investigation*, Institute for the Study of Labor IZA DP No. 1758 (September 2005).

70. For example, James Heyman and Dan Ariely found that when students were surveyed about how likely they thought it would be that other students would help load a couch into a van they believed that more people would when no monetary incentive was offered than would help when only a small incentive was offered. "Effort for Payment: A Tale of Two Markets," *Psychological Science* 15, 11 (2004), 789. Similarly, Felix Warneken and Michael Tomasello found that 20-month-old children were keen to help an adult retrieve an object that was out of reach but when they were rewarded with a toy for their effort the rate at which they were willing to help fell significantly. "Extrinsic Rewards Undermine Altruistic Tendencies in 20-Month-Olds," *Developmental Psychology* 44, 6 (2008), 1785–1788.

71. WHO, *Towards Self-Sufficiency in Safe Blood and Blood Products*, 5.

72. J.D. Jasper et al. were here writing of the possible effects that compensation would have on the number of transplant organs that would be procured but their point can readily be generalized to the same question posed for plasma. "Altruism, Incentives, and Organ Donation Attitudes of the Transplant Community," *Medical Care* 42, 4 (2004), 384.

73. This was noted in the Introduction to this volume.

74. M.P. Janssen, L.R. van Hoeven, and G. Rautmann, *Trends and Observations on the Collection, Testing and Use of Blood and Blood Components in Europe 2001–2011 Report* (Strasbourg: European Directorate for the Quality of Medicines & HealthCare of the Council of Europe [EDQM], 2015), 27. The Czech Republic is especially interesting. As Grabowski and Manning note, in 2001, "the Czech Republic provided plasma at among the lowest rates in Europe." After it allowed donor compensation in 2007, by 2011 "it was providing plasma at more than double the rate per capita of most other European countries." "An Economic Analysis of Global Policy Proposals to Prohibit Compensation of Blood Plasma Donors," 158.

75. Austria – which allows donor compensation – did not report data for 2011. However, in 2010 it collected 12.45 L of plasma for fractionation per 1000 inhabitants (Janssen et al., *Trends and Observations*, 27). This datum does

not undermine the claim that the offer of compensation leads to an increase in the amount of plasma collected in comparison to a situation in which compensation is prohibited. Instead, it simply underscores that compensation alone will not lead to an increase in the volume of plasma procured; there must also be the infrastructure in place to collect plasma.

76. Ibid.
77. 23,730 L of plasma for fractionation were collected in the United States in 2012. Patrick Robert, "Self-Sufficiency: Facts and Pitfalls!" *The Source* (Fall 2014), 35. The population of the United States was c. 315,091,138 on January 1, 2013. (United States Census Bureau (CB12–255), Available at: www.census.gov/newsroom/releases/archives/population/cb12-255.html).
78. Mark Weinstein, "Regulation of plasma for fractionation in the United States," *Annals of Blood* 2, 3 (2018), 8, Table 7. Germany permits 45 and the UK permits 24.
79. Ibid. Note that these figures refer to the volume of plasma collected; the overall permissible collection volume is higher (e.g., 880 mL for 800 mL of plasma collected). See the FDA memorandum "Volume Limits – Automated Collection of Source Plasma" dated November 4, 1992, 1. (This memo was cited by Alan E. Williams, who, in turn, was cited by Weinstein; see note 81.)
80. The United States figure of 800 mL, for example, applies only to donors who weigh at least 175 lb; a donor who weighs between 150 and 174 lb can only donate 750 mL of plasma per donation, while a donor who weighs between 110 and 149 lb can only donate 625 nL per donation. See Alan E. Williams, "FDA Considerations Regarding Frequent Plasma Collection Procedures," *15th International Haemovigilance Seminar, Brussels, Belgium*. Available at: www.ihn-org.com/wp-content/ slide 8. Williams is here referring to "Volume Limits – Automated Collection of Source Plasma."
81. Weinstein, "Regulation of Plasma for Fractionation in the United States," 8. Weinstein here cites Williams, "FDA Considerations Regarding Frequent Plasma Collection Procedures," who, in turn, provides a figure of 63–83 L a year for the United States and 29–38 L a year for Germany. See Williams, "FDA Considerations Regarding Frequent Plasma Collection Procedures," slide 9.
82. George Brooks Schreiber and Mary Clare Kimber, "Source Plasma Donors: A Snapshot," *Poster Presented AABB Annual Meeting; San Diego, CA* (October 7–10, 2017). Available at: www.pptaglobal.org/images/presentations/2017/Schreiber.AABBposterAbstract_Source_Plasma_Donors_A_Snapshot_2017_9.27.17.pdf
83. All of these data are from Schreiber and Kimber, "Source Plasma Donors."
84. Uri Gneezy and Aldo Rustichini, "Pay Enough – or don't Pay at All," *The Quarterly Journal of Economics* 115, 3 (2000), 791–810. See also Uri Gneezy, Stephan Meier, and Pedro Rey-Biel, "When and Why Incentives (Don't) Work to Modify Behavior," *Journal of Economic Perspectives* 25, 4 (Fall 2011), 193, and Gneezy and Rustichini, "A Fine Is a Price," 15.
85. Note that this is still a legitimate concern even if the majority of donors in the United States do not take full advantage of the opportunities that they have to donate.
86. J. Pink, B. Bell, G. Kotsiou, S. Wright, and J. Thyer, "Safe and Sustainable Plasmapheresis," *ISBT Science Series* 12, 4 (2017), 471–472.
87. These concerns were noted, but not endorsed, by T. Schulzki et al., "A Prospective Multicentre Study on the Safety of Long-Term Intensive Plasmapheresis in Donors (SIPLA)," *Vox Sanguinis* 91 (2006), 163.

88. George B. Schreiber, Roger Brinser, Marilyn Rosa-Bray, Zi-Fan Yu, and Toby Simon, "Frequent Source Plasma Donors are not at Risk of Iron Depletion: The Ferritin Levels in Plasma Donor (FLIPD) study," *Transfusion* 58 (2018), 951, 958.
89. M. Rodell, "Collection of Source Material from Remunerated Donors," *Developments in Biological Standardization* 81 (1993), 57–64.
90. M.B. Rodell and M.L. Lee, "Determination of Reasons for Cessation of Participation in Serial Plasmapheresis Programs," *Transfusion* 39 (1999), 901.
91. Ibid., 902.
92. S. Bechtloff, B. Tran-My, H. Haubelt, G. Stelzer, C. Anders, and P. Hellstern, "A Prospective Trial on the Safety of Long-Term Intensive Plasmapheresis in Donors," *Vox Sanguinis* 88 (2005), 189–195.
93. Ibid., 189.
94. Ibid., 190.
95. Ibid.
96. Ibid., 194. It is also much higher than the average of 17.5 donations a year (in 2012) reported by Schreiber and Kimber.
97. Ibid.
98. Ibid.
99. Ibid.
100. Ibid.
101. Ibid., 195.
102. Ibid.
103. T. Schulzki, "A Prospective Multicentre Study on the Safety of Long-Term Intensive Plasmapheresis in Donors (SIPLA)," 163.

2 Donor Compensation and Informed Consent

Introduction

I argued in the previous chapter that not only were the empirical concerns voiced by the defenders of prohibiting donor compensation mistaken, they were also misguided: Persons genuinely concerned with patient health should support donor compensation not oppose it. This chapter will proceed similarly, taking as its starting point one of the claims addressed in the last chapter: That donor compensation will crowd out some prospective plasma donors leading to a decrease in the overall amount of plasma procured. As was previously discussed, this claim is false. There is evidence that some prospective plasma donors would be deterred from donating if a low level of compensation is offered. However, there is also considerable evidence that increasing the amount of compensation would rectify this. Indeed, there is significant evidence that offering a reasonable amount of compensation (e.g., $35 a donation) will secure considerably more plasma than would be secured where no compensation is to be offered at all.

These instrumental concerns are not, however, the focus of this chapter. Instead, I will establish an interesting *ethical* conclusion: That offers of compensation are *required* to enable some donors to give their informed consent to donate. I will argue that the need to offer donor compensation for this reason is supported by the evidence that offers of low levels of compensation can undermine some prospective donors' motivation to donate. Offers of compensation provide information to prospective donors concerning the economic value of their donation. Once they have this information, some donors reconsider their original intention to donate. These empirical claims are then combined with an ethical axiom that is widely accepted by medical professionals, bioethicists, and moral philosophers who work on bioethics: That (if possible) persons should give their informed consent to any medical procedures that they undergo. This combination leads to the conclusion that to protect prospective donors' ability to give their informed consent to the donation of

DOI: 10.4324/9781003263913-3

their plasma, plasma centers should not be prohibited from offering them compensation.

This chapter consists of five sections. In the first, I will outline an account of the conditions that must be met for a person to give her informed consent to the medical procedures that she is subject to. I will note that the core element of healthcare professionals' duty to secure the informed consent of their patients to their treatment is the obligation to disclose information that is relevant to their patients' treatment decisions. The question of which information counts as relevant in this context is admittedly controversial. However, the controversy over the requirements that the doctrine of informed consent places upon healthcare professionals is immaterial to the main argument of this chapter. The two most defensible standards by which the relevance of information could be assessed – the "reasonable person standard" and the "subjective standard" – both support the conclusion that the ethical requirement to secure patients' informed consent to their medical treatment requires that plasma centers be allowed to offer compensation to donors.[1] In the second section of this chapter, I provide evidence for the claim that some levels of compensation will lead to a reduction in the amount of plasma that is procured by "crowding out" (i.e., deterring) more donors than would be "crowded in" (i.e., motivated to donate) by the offer of compensation. The purpose of this section is not to engage with the debate over the effects that offers of compensation would have on the amount of plasma procured – a debate whose conclusions are in any case settled.[2] Instead, it is to establish two claims. First, that for some potential donors the question of *whether* compensation is offered for the donation of plasma is relevant to their decision as to whether or not to donate. Second, that for some donors the *amount* of compensation that is offered is relevant to their decision as to whether or not to donate. I will then argue in the third section of this chapter that those persons for whom information about the amount of compensation that is (or would be) offered for donating plasma is relevant to their decisions as to whether or not to donate would only be able to give their informed consent to donate plasma when compensation is offered. Thus, I will argue, a moral concern with securing donors' informed consent to donate their plasma requires that plasma centers be allowed to offer them compensation. In the fourth and fifth sections of this chapter, I will outline and respond to objections, both to the argument that I develop in this chapter and to the general argumentative approach that I have adopted.

Informed Consent and the Requirement to Disclose

As Beauchamp and Childress note in their seminal work, *Principles of Biomedical Ethics*, "biomedical ethics has placed consent at the forefront of its concerns" since the exposure at the Nuremburg trials of the

Nazis' medical experiments.[3] In the context of the donation of blood and blood products, the need for *informed* consent is expressly endorsed by the International Society of Blood Transfusion, who have enshrined it in the first Clause of their Code of Ethics: "[t]he donor should provide informed consent to the donation of blood or blood components."[4] There is debate over whether the primary justification for the need to secure a person's informed consent to her medical treatment should be grounded on a moral concern for the value of her autonomy, or a moral concern for the value of her well-being.[5] There is, however, still broad agreement (at least within the West) that the bioethical concern with informed consent focuses on the ethical requirement that a person should autonomously authorize the treatment to which she is subject.[6] This naturally leads to the question of what conditions must be met for a person autonomously to authorize her treatment. There is considerable debate over this issue both within the literature on personal autonomy and within the litera- ture on informed consent.[7] However, all parties to this debate – whether they are autonomy theorists who are concerned with analyzing what conditions must be met for a person to be autonomous with respect to her actions, or bioethicists who are concerned with offering analyses of informed consent – agree that for a person to give her informed consent to a procedure the healthcare professionals who are treating her should disclose the information that is material to her decision.

Autonomy theorists agree that to be autonomous a person must be *self-ruled*.[8] To the extent that the actions that a person performs are deter- mined by another, then, she will undergo a diminution in her autonomy with respect to them. Hence, if a healthcare professional intentionally fails to disclose information with the aim of influencing his patient's deci- sion in a particular way, then to the extent that he is successful in this, it will be he, and not she, who is directing her actions. As such, she will undergo a diminution in her autonomy with respect to the actions that she consequently performs. Thus, for autonomy theorists, for a person to autonomously authorize her treatment she must have authorized it without having been led to do so by her healthcare provider's intentional failure to disclose information, where this failure to disclose resulted in her making a decision that she would not have made had she had access to the information in question.[9]

Informed Consent in Autonomy Theory and Bioethics

Analyses of what is required for a person to give her informed consent that have been developed by bioethicists similarly focus on healthcare providers' duty to disclose information that is relevant to their patient's decision. This duty to disclose is central to accounts of informed con- sent that have been developed in the medical literature, the policy litera- ture, and the philosophical literature.[10] This is not surprising. If informed consent is construed to be synonymous with a person's autonomously authorizing her treatment, then the conditions that must be met for a person to give her informed consent should track those that have been identified in the autonomy literature as those that must be met for her to be autonomous with respect to her authorizing action. However, the focus on disclosure within those accounts of informed consent that have been developed in the bioethics literature differs from that within those developed by autonomy theorists in one important respect: They focus on the requirement that healthcare professionals disclose relevant information to their patients *simpliciter* rather than merely attempting to preclude *intentional* nondisclosure. This, too, is not surprising. The analyses of informed consent that have been developed in the literature on autonomy are primarily focused on the *theoretical* question of whether a person is autonomous with respect to her authorizing act. The answer to this will be determined by whether or not her performance of this act meets certain theoretical conditions. The question of whether one could tell *in practice* if a person's authorizing act met these conditions is not of immediate concern to autonomy theorists. That it might be impossible in many cases to tell whether a healthcare professional's failure to disclose relevant information to a patient was intentional or not would thus not be of concern to them. By contrast, accounts of informed consent that have been developed within the bioethics literature are intended to be applicable *in practice*. They thus tend to avoid offering conditions for informed consent whose satisfaction would be difficult to determine. For the (practical) bioethical approach to informed consent, the primary question is hence not whether a healthcare professional *intentionally* failed to disclose relevant information to her patient but simply whether she failed to meet the standards that govern the disclosure of relevant information.

Clarifying the relationship between the accounts of informed consent that have been developed in the theoretical literature on autonomy and those that have been developed in the bioethical literature is both interesting and important. However, for the purposes of this chapter, it is important only to note that both approaches to informed consent have at their core the requirement that healthcare professionals disclose to their patients information that is relevant to the decisions that they are faced with.

Information Relevant to Informed Consent

What information, then, should be taken to be relevant to a patient's decision for the purpose of assessing whether she has given her informed consent? There are (at least) three possible answers to this question. The first, the "professional practice" standard, is that the information relevant to a patient's decision is that which is judged to be relevant by healthcare professionals.[11] The second, the "reasonable person" (or "prudent patient") standard, holds that the information that should be disclosed to the patient is that which a "reasonable person" would want to be disclosed to her.[12] The final answer to the question of what information should be taken to be relevant to a patient's decision, and hence disclosed to her so that she can give her informed consent to her treatment procedure, is the "subjective standard." On this approach, the information that should be deemed to be relevant to a person's decisions concerning her treatment should be determined by the specific interests of the patient in question in receiving certain information.

Of these three standards for disclosure, the professional practice standard is beset by the most practical and theoretical difficulties. First, it is not clear that there exists a uniform professional standard for disclosure of the sort that it presupposes.[13] Second, even if such a standard did exist it might still fall far short of that which would be required for a person genuinely autonomously to authorize a course of treatment. Indeed, the professional practice standard is compatible with the systematic usurpation of patient autonomy by healthcare professionals through a widespread and deliberate failure to disclose certain information with the aim of directing patients to choose one type of treatment over another.[14] Third, since this standard of disclosure is indexed to the professional practice of healthcare professionals it would likely focus upon the disclosure of information pertaining to the medical effects of treatment. However, patients will have other concerns besides their medical interests that would affect the decisions that they make concerning their treatment options – and these might be ignored if the professional practice standard of disclosure is adopted. Finally, even if the professional practice standard was created in an attempt to serve the best interests of patients all things considered (and not merely their perceived medical interests) healthcare professionals *qua* healthcare professionals do not have any privileged position in assessing where these interests lie. Accordingly, in adopting this model they would be imposing their view of what is in their patients' interests onto them. It would thus be they who would, in part, be directing their patients' decisions – and to the extent that this is so they would compromise their patients' autonomy. The professional practice standard of disclosure is thus self-defeating.

There is, then, good reason to reject the professional practice standard of disclosure. However, both the reasonable person standard and the subjective standard also face difficulties. The reasonable person standard faces the obvious problem that it is too vague to be readily applicable, for it is not clear what information a "reasonable" or "prudent" patient would require. Moreover, just as on the professional practice standard there could be a gap between the information that it requires to be disclosed to patients and the information that particular patients would need to give their informed consent, so too is it likely that "[t]he individual patient will have interests and needs which might bear little relationship to the 'prudent patient' however conceptualized."[15] The natural solution to this problem is to move to the subjective standard where the information that should be disclosed to a patient will be indexed to her particular interests. Unfortunately, the very subjectivity of this standard renders it difficult to apply in practice. It would require healthcare professionals to "do an exhaustive background and character analysis of each patient to determine the relevant information" for her.[16] Moreover, it could be the case that patients (and hence healthcare professionals) would only know what information would be relevant to their medical decisions after they have undergone treatment and fully understand the implications of its effects.

Yet while all three accounts of which information should be disclosed to patients to secure their informed consent to their treatment face difficulties, those that are faced by the reasonable person standard and the subjective standard differ in kind from those that are faced by the professional practice standard. The objections to the professional practice standard focus on showing why its application would be likely to fail to secure a patient's autonomous authorization of her course of treatment, and why, instead, it could lead to the usurpation of a patient's autonomy by the healthcare professionals who are treating her. The concerns about the reasonable person standard and the subjective standard, however, focus only on how practically applicable these approaches could be in identifying what information should be disclosed to patients. This type of objection leaves open the possibility that in some situations it will be clear both what information the reasonable person standard would require be disclosed to would-be donors, and also what information it is likely that the subjective standard would require be disclosed to them.[17] As I will argue later, this will be the case when persons are considering donating plasma. The behavior of some uncompensated donors when compensation is introduced supports the view that the reasonable person standard would require that potential donors be informed of the possibility of receiving compensation for their donation. And, I will argue, for many would-be donors, the subjective standard would support this disclosure also. From this, I will argue that the reasonable person standard would require, and the subjective standard would likely require, that to give their informed consent to donation prospective plasma donors should be informed of the amount of offered compensation that would be offered for their donations.

Crowding Out and Compensated Donation

As I noted in Chapter 1, there is some empirical evidence that some offers of compensation will lead to lower donation rates of blood and blood products.[18] I will outline this evidence here – but not to provide support for the (false) claim that allowing compensated donation will reduce the amount of plasma collected. Instead, I outline the evidence that some offers of compensation will deter some potential donors from donating their plasma to lay the groundwork for the claim that the reasonable person standard of disclosure would require, and the subjective standard of disclosure would likely require, that to give their informed consent to donation prospective plasma donors should be informed of the amount of compensation that would be offered for their donations.

The crowding-out arguments against compensated donation begin with the claim that when compensation is introduced into a situation where the donors of plasma (or other body parts) were previously uncompensated, some donors will either be deterred from donating, or, if they are already donating, will cease to do so. This claim is supported by a study conducted by Mellstrom and Johannesson in Sweden.[19] (That this study was conducted on potential blood donors, rather than potential plasma donors, makes no difference to the argument concerning compensation and informed consent that follows.) Prior to donating blood in Sweden potential donors are required to undergo a health examination. In Mellstrom and Johannesson's experiment, three different approaches to secure persons willing to undergo this examination were taken. (Mellstrom and Johannesson only attempted to secure persons to agree to undergo the health examination who had not yet undergone the health examination and who were not already aware that they could not be blood donors as they met exclusion criteria.)[20] In the first "no payment" approach, no compensation was offered to subjects to complete this examination. In the second approach ("SEK 50 payment"), persons were offered SEK 50 (about $7) to complete the examination. In the third approach ("SEK 50 payment with charity option"), persons could choose between receiving the SEK 50 themselves or donating this amount to charity.

Mellstrom and Johannesson found that of the (male and female) subjects that were approached with no offer of payment, 43% agreed to become blood donors, while of those who were offered payment only 33% agreed. This latter number increased to 44% when the option to donate to charity was introduced.[21] They also found that when these results were disaggregated by gender there was a marked difference between the responses of men and women, with women evincing a "sizeable" crowding-out effect. When the "SEK 50 payment" option was offered to women, the percentage of subjects who would agree to donate blood dropped from 52% to 30%. However, when they were offered the "SEK 50 payment with charity option," this crowding-out effect was counteracted and the percentage of subjects willing to donate rose to 53%.[22]

Mellstrom and Johannesson conclude from this data that "the skepticism towards monetary compensation for blood donations . . . is warranted."[23] (And so, by implication, is the similar skepticism toward monetary compensation for plasma donations.) I have already addressed the question of whether such skepticism is warranted in Chapter 1, and I will address it again later. Before I do so, however, I will discuss the implications of Mellstrom's and Johannesson's results for the requirement that persons give their informed consent to donating plasma.

Compensated Donation, Crowding Out, and Informed Consent

Mellstrom's and Johannesson's study shows clearly that some donors are deterred from donating blood (and, by extrapolation, plasma), once compensation is offered. While the motivations for such cessation of donation will no doubt vary an economic analysis of why some people would cease to donate when compensation is offered yields important implications for the debate over the ethics of compensating plasma donors.[24]

A person's decision not to donate plasma could indicate that, to her, the opportunity costs of donating are higher than the value that she places on her act of donation. If a person uses the degree of compensation that she is offered to donate as a proxy for the value of her donation, then if the amount of compensation offered is lower than the opportunity costs that she believes that she will incur in donating, she will not donate. The explanation of why such a person would cease donating (or would be deterred from donating) once compensation was offered when she willingly donated (or was willing to donate) prior to this is simple.[25] Prior to the offer of compensation, she believed that the value of her donation was greater than the opportunity costs that she perceived herself incurring to donate. However, once compensation was offered – and given that she used the level of compensation offered as a proxy for the value of her donation – she came to believe that the value of her donation was lower than the opportunity costs that she believed that she incurred in making it. As such, then, once compensation was offered, she would cease to donate. To illustrate this, consider a person who earns SEK 100 an hour and who routinely spends an hour of her time donating plasma in a situation where no compensation for donation was offered. This person donates because she believes that the value of her donation to its proximate recipients was greater than SEK 100, and so she believes that her time was better spent donating plasma than working to earn SEK 100. However, if compensation is introduced at the rate of SEK 50 per plasma donation, then (holding the time spend on donating plasma constant) this person would now learn that her donation was worth less (SEK 50) than the time that she would have to spend donating (SEK 100). In this situation, it would be better if she did *not* donate her plasma.[26] The opportunity costs of such donation (SEK 100) would be greater than its benefits (SEK 50). Thus, once compensation is offered donors whose opportunity costs of donation would exceed the level of compensation that they are offered *should* cease to donate.[27] Their donations *should* be crowded out by the level of compensation that is offered.

Why Informed Consent Requires Donor Compensation

This analysis of why some plasma donors would cease to donate once compensation is offered can be used to show that to satisfy the ethical requirement of securing persons' informed consent to the medical procedures that they undergo there should be no prohibition on the offer of compensation to plasma donors.

The aforementioned analysis is based on the view that if the degree of compensation that is offered to secure a good or service is lower than the perceived opportunity cost of providing it, a rational person will not provide the good or service in question.[28] The degree of compensation that is offered for a good or a service will be a function of the demand for it together with its supply. Since demand for plasma is relatively inelastic, the level of compensation that will need to be offered to secure a sufficient supply of it will be primarily driven by the amount that is being supplied. If too little is being supplied, then the level of compensation offered will rise; if too much, then the level of compensation offered will fall. The amount of plasma that is supplied at any given time will thus be a function of two variables: (1) the costs to the donors that are associated with providing it, such as the time spent in the plasma center, the time spent getting to the plasma center, and the experiences that are associated with donating and (2) the level of compensation that is offered to offset these costs. Assume that the time spent providing plasma and the experiences in the plasma centers will be relatively comparable for all donors. If this is so, then the primary variable which will distinguish between persons who would donate plasma given a particular level of compensation offered and those who would not do so will be determined by their relative perceived opportunity costs. Since this is so, given the inelasticity of the demand for plasma, the level of compensation offered for it will be determined by the opportunity costs of donating that would be incurred by the donors. That is, the level of compensation that would need to be offered to plasma donors will indicate the highest boundary of opportunity cost that needs to be compensated for to secure the amount of plasma that is in demand. A prospective plasma donor who uses the degree of compensation that she is offered to donate plasma as a proxy for the value of her act of donation and who only wishes to donate when the value of her donation would exceed her opportunity costs could thus tell from the amount of compensation that is offered whether she should donate or whether she should leave donation to others.[29] If the level of compensation offered is greater than her perceived opportunity costs of donating, then she should donate. If it is lower, then she should leave the donation of plasma to others (i.e., who perceive their opportunity costs to be lower).[30] To make this assessment, a prospective plasma donor needs to know only two things: Her own opportunity costs and the level of compensation that is being offered for her plasma. For such a would-be donor to make an informed decision about whether she should donate plasma or leave this to someone else, she must be able to have access to information about the level of compensation that is being offered for plasma at the time she is considering donating. If plasma donors are not compensated, such a donor would lack information that could have been crucial to her making an informed decision about whether or not to donate.

Compensation, Signaling, and Charitable Donations

This analysis of why some donors would be crowded out by the offer of compensation supports the view that the need to secure donors' informed consent to donating requires that compensation for their donations not be prohibited. Before moving to defend this view, I will note that it is compatible with Mellstrom and Johannesson's data showing that female blood donors were crowded out by the "SEK 50 payment" but were crowded *in* by the "SEK 50 payment with charity option." This is important. On the face of it, the differential response of some of the female subjects in this study to these two offers would appear to contradict the earlier analysis. Since these offers have the same economic value if the earlier analysis was correct then it might appear that subjects who were crowded out by the "SEK 50 payment" (as this was lower than their opportunity costs of donating) should *also* be crowded out by the "SEK 50 payment with charity option." But this overlooks the possibility that these female subjects might value using their non-compensated donation of blood to signal others how charitable they are at more than SEK 50. If this is so, then they would donate blood for no payment as the value of the signal that they could send by so doing was worth more to them than the opportunity costs that they would incur by donating. However, they would *not* donate blood for a payment of SEK 50 as such a payment would both be of lower value to them than the signal that they could send in its absence, *and* it would be lower than the opportunity costs that they would incur by donating. Such subjects would, however, donate blood if they were offered the "SEK 50 payment with charity option," for then they would again secure the value of signaling how charitable they were which is greater than their opportunity costs of donating. (Indeed, if the donation of blood and the SEK 50 payment would be a more effective signal than only the donation of blood – and hence would be more valuable as such – it is to be expected that more persons with the desire to signal their charitableness would be willing to donate blood as a greater number of such persons could have their opportunity costs bought out by the greater value of this enhanced signal.) The earlier analysis of why some donors are crowded out by the offer of compensation is thus fully compatible with Mellstrom and Johannesson's experimental results.

The Irrelevance of Economic Value for Some Donors

I argued previously that for some prospective donors to be able to make informed decisions about whether or not to donate plasma they must have access to information about the level of compensation that is being offered for plasma at the time they are considering donating. For such donors, then, it is clear that the subjective standard of disclosure would require both that compensation for their donations be available to them and that information about the amount of compensation on offer be available to them for them to give their informed consent to the donation of their plasma.[31] (I will argue later that the reasonable person standard of disclosure also supports offering donor compensation.) However, not all donors would desire to know whether the value of their donation exceeded their opportunity costs of donating. Some donors might, for example, wish to donate to signal their charitable nature and would donate plasma independently of the value of their donations as such an act is a socially recognized means of signaling that one is charitable. Others might donate simply because they believe that they are morally obligated to do so, or because they feel a "warm glow" of pleasure from the donation that they cannot achieve any other way. For these donors, the economic value of their donation plays no role in their deliberation over whether or not to donate. Recognizing the existence of such donors is important for the argument that is being developed here. It shows that this argument can acknowledge without loss of force the fact that there are many activities that persons engage in without knowing the level of compensation that they would be offered to perform them without this lack of information making their engagement in these activities any less consensual. For example, if a person does not care how much his partner would pay him to have sex with her that he does not know how much she might pay him to perform it does not thereby render their lovemaking any less consensual if this information is of no concern to him. Similarly, a wealthy woman's act of giving away her art collection to a museum would not be any less consensual if she did this without knowing how much each piece would fetch at auction if their financial value would not affect her motivation to donate them.

But that not all prospective donors would desire to know the economic value of their donation does not undermine the claim that respecting the need to secure donors' informed consent to donating plasma requires that they not be prohibited from being offered compensation for their donations, and that they be informed of the amount of compensation on offer. Even though not all prospective donors would need to be informed of the economic value of their plasma donations to give their informed consent to donate, it is likely that some would. To secure the informed consent of those donors compensation must be offered to them, with the amount that is offered being clear. The need to offer compensation to these donors to provide them with the economic information required for them to give their informed consent to donate would be endorsed by persons who adhere to the subjective standard for the disclosure of information to secure her informed consent. However, it would not be possible to identify *a priori* those donors who would need to know the economic value of their donation to give their informed consent to donate. Compensation should accordingly be offered to *all* prospective donors to ensure that those for whom information about the economic value of their donation that the level of compensation offered would provide would receive the information that they require to give their informed consent. It is thus reasonable to require that compensation be offered to all prospective donors. It would thus be reasonable for a prospective donor to expect that she would be offered compensation. This being so, on the reasonable person standard of information that should be disclosed so that persons can provide their informed consent to the medical procedures that they undergo, prospective donors should be offered compensation. The level of compensation that would be offered would provide them with information that a reasonable person would expect to receive prior to making her decision as to whether or not to consent to donate. Thus, both the subjective standard and the reasonable person standard for determining the information that should be provided to a person so that she can give her informed consent to her treatment require that compensation be offered to prospective donors so that they would have the appropriate level of information that they need to give their informed consent to their donation.[32] The moral need to secure donors' informed consent thus requires that they be offered compensation for their donations.

Objections and Responses

The earlier argument faces two serious objections. The proponents of these objections accept that the earlier argument is sound and so prospective plasma donors should not be precluded from having the information concerning the economic value of their donation that the offer of compensation can provide them with. However, the proponent of the first objection charges, this information could be provided to potential donors through the offer of *hypothetical*, rather than *actual*, compensation. The ethical obligation to provide information to the typical prospective donor about the level of compensation that would be offered for her donation could be discharged simply by informing potential donors of what the amount *would have* been. No actual compensation needs to be given. The proponent of the second objection also denies that prospective plasma donors should be offered actual compensation. Compensation need not be offered provided that donors were drawn only from the ranks of those for whom information about the level of compensation that they would receive for their donation is not relevant to their decision to donate.

The First Objection

The first objection is initially plausible. However, it rests on the assumption that the amount of compensation that needs to be offered by collection agencies to prospective donors to secure the amount of plasma that is required could be known even if no actual compensation was offered. This assumption is false. Recall that since the demand for plasma is relatively inelastic the level of compensation that plasma centers will need to offer potential donors to secure what is needed will primarily depend on prospective donors' opportunity costs. The plasma centers could never ascertain what these costs are unless they had an accurate way of securing this information from the members of the pool of potential donors. They could not secure this information from their would-be donors through means of polling. Prospective donors' perceived opportunity costs would constantly be in flux and a poll could only provide a snapshot of the opportunity costs that would be incurred at a particular point in time. There would also be no guarantee that a poll could provide an accurate account of donors' perceived opportunity costs at a particular point in time, for the opportunity costs that the polled would-be donors claimed they believed they would incur might be inaccurate. (Most obviously, they would have an incentive to inflate the opportunity costs that they would claim to incur to try to raise the level of compensation that would be offered.) The only accurate means by which the plasma centers could tell what the requisite level of compensation would need to be offered for them to secure the amount of plasma that they needed would be *actually* to offer compensation for it. If the amount of compensation offered was lower than the higher boundary of opportunity costs that needed to be compensated for to secure the requisite amount of plasma, then too little plasma would be secured. If it were higher than this boundary, then more potential donors would offer their plasma than would be needed. On receiving this information, the plasma centers could adjust the level of compensation that they offered until they arrived at an equilibrium between the amount of plasma that they needed and the amount that was donated. (Although this equilibrium would be unstable owing to the ever-fluctuating opportunity costs of the potential donors.) The ethical obligation to provide prospective donors with accurate information about the level of compensation that plasma collection agencies would need to offer to secure the requisite amount of plasma could thus only be discharged by the offer of *actual* compensation.

The Second Objection

The aforementioned response assumes that prospective donors would need to know the actual level of compensation that they would be offered for their plasma to give their informed consent to donation. But this would not be the case for those donors for whom information about the level of compensation that they would be offered for their plasma is not relevant to their deliberations as to whether or not to donate. The earlier argument that the need to secure donors' informed consent to their plasma donations requires that they be offered compensation is thus compatible with two conclusions. It is, clearly, compatible with the conclusion that compensation should be offered to prospective donors so that they can give their informed consent to donate their plasma. But it is *also* compatible with the conclusion that *no* compensation needs to be offered to donors. This would be the case if prospective donors were screened to identify those who would not be concerned with the level of compensation that would be offered for their donations and for donations only to be accepted from these donors. Under this system, plasma donations would only be accepted from persons for whom information about the economic value of their donation would be irrelevant to their decision to donate. Since this is so the donors from whom plasma was accepted in this system could give their informed consent to donate even in the absence of compensation. This system of plasma procurement could operate in conjunction with a prohibition on donor compensation. The earlier argument has thus not established that a concern for securing donors' informed consent leads to the ethical requirement that there should be no prohibition on compensation being offered to plasma donors.

This is certainly a powerful objection. However, it only succeeds as an objection to the argument that prospective donors must be offered compensation if it posits *both* that donors be screened so that plasma is only procured from those who take no interest in the economic value of their donation *and* that this system operates in conjunction with the prohibition of donor compensation. It is not an objection to the earlier (pro-compensation) argument to note that a prospective donor's informed consent to her donation can be secured even if she has no knowledge of its economic value provided that this information is not relevant to her decision. This possibility is perfectly compatible with its conclusion that donors should not be prohibited from receiving compensation. This second objection must thus support a "screened donor, no compensation" system of plasma procurement if it is to function as an objection to the requirement that donors be offered compensation. But since this is so the levels of plasma that the system required by this objection would procure would be lower than those procured in a system where donor compensation was allowed.[33] Moreover, given that this "screened donor, no compensation" system of plasma procurement would procure plasma *only* from persons who took no interest in the economic value of their donation it would be likely to secure even *less* plasma than do the current systems of uncompensated plasma procurement. The current systems of plasma procurement that prohibit donor compensation procure plasma both from persons who take no interest in its economic value *and* from persons who would take its economic value into account when deciding whether or not to donate if this information were available to them.[34] Screening out the latter group of donors would thus result in less plasma being procured. And if the reduced amount of plasma collected would be insufficient to meet medical needs, this will have an adverse effect on patient well-being compared to a situation where donor compensation is not prohibited.

This response could function as an independent consequentialist response to this objection. (In this role, it would hold that the "screened donor, no compensation" model would lead to less well-being than a procurement system that allowed donor compensation.) However, (and more importantly for this discussion) it also functions as a response that is concerned with the moral importance of securing a person's informed consent to her treatment. It does so in the same way that another response to this second objection works against it – one that is based on the moral value of personal autonomy. (Consider this as a promissory note.) To show this, I will briefly outline how the "screened donor, no compensation" approach will compromise the autonomy of some prospective donors (and some persons who operate plasma centers).

As I noted earlier for the "screened donor, no compensation" model to function as an objection to the earlier pro-compensation argument, it would have to be conjoined with a prohibition on donor compensation. As I will argue more fully in Chapter 3 to prohibit donor compensation is to attempt to coerce prospective donors who would wish to receive compensation for their plasma donations and persons who would wish to compensate them for donating from transacting. If this prohibition successfully precludes such transactions, then the persons who would have otherwise engaged in them would have been successfully coerced into refraining from so doing. Successfully subjecting a person to coercion would result in the actions that she performed being determined (at least in part) by another (namely, her coercer). Since this is so then a person who was coerced would suffer from a diminution in her autonomy with respect to her actions. Thus, given the moral importance that is accorded to autonomy within contemporary (Western) bioethics, there is at least *prima facie* reason to morally oppose the prohibition of compensated donation.[35]

As with the earlier consequentialist response, this autonomy-based response could function as an independent response to the second objection. (In this role it would hold that the moral wrong of compromising the autonomy of those adversely affected by the prohibition on donor compensation would render the "screened donor, no compensation" model wrongful.) But as with the first (well-being-based) response to this second objection, it also functions as a response that is concerned with the moral importance of securing a person's informed consent to her medical treatment. It is now time to pay off the promissory note I issued earlier and explain how both a moral concern for well-being and a moral concern for autonomy both function as responses concerned with the moral importance of securing a person's informed consent to her treatment.

The moral concern with informed consent is not based on the value of securing a person's informed consent to her treatment for its own sake. Rather, it is based on a moral concern with either the well-being or (and more typically) the autonomy of the person whose informed consent is sought.[36] A system of plasma procurement that would result in lower well-being than alternative systems and that would compromise persons' autonomy should not be supported by those who believe that there is a moral requirement to secure a person's informed consent to her medical treatment. Hence, while a system of "screened donor, no compensation" would be able to secure the informed consent of its screened donors, the moral concern with the values of well-being and autonomy that undergird the moral importance of informed consent would not support it. Thus, insofar as a concern for informed consent evinces a concern for one (or both) of these morally important properties one who believes that securing a person's informed consent to her treatment should oppose this system of plasma procurement even though it is still narrowly compatible with securing the informed consent of its donors.

Well-Being, Autonomy, and Donor Compensation

This response to the second objection leads to one final issue that must be addressed in this chapter. Since a concern for the moral value of either well-being or autonomy supports both the ethical requirement to secure a person's informed consent to her treatment and the conclusion that donor compensation should not be prohibited, why should not these values be drawn upon directly to argue for the latter conclusion? That is, why need one argue for the view that a moral concern for informed consent supports the view that donor compensation should not be prohibited if the conclusion that it should not be prohibited could be derived more directly by appeal to the ethical values that undergird the requirement to secure a person's informed consent?

There are three responses that can be given to this question. First, that the amount of compensation that donors would be offered for their plasma conveys information that would be relevant to some persons' decisions as to whether or not to donate has until now been overlooked in the literatures both on informed consent and on the ethics of donor compensation. This chapter corrects this serious omission. Second, this chapter shows that the evidence that some donors are crowded out by the offer of payment (such as that presented by Mellstrom and Johannesson) does not necessarily support the view that donors should not be offered compensation. Instead, it supports the view that donors *should* be offered compensation if we are concerned about their ability to give their informed consent to donate. Some donors might have been crowded out by the offer of compensation as this offer presented them with information about the economic value of their donation that they previously lacked, and that was relevant to their decision concerning whether or not to donate. Finally – and perhaps most importantly – the ethical requirement to secure a person's informed consent to her treatment is both widely accepted within bioethics and widely enshrined in law.[37] Demonstrating that a practical approach to plasma procurement would require offering compensation to prospective donors to ensure that they can provide their informed consent to their donation is a direct means to demonstrate that donor compensation is ethically required – and that its prohibition is unethical.

Conclusion

I noted in the Introduction to this volume that the debate over donor compensation has taken a now-familiar form: The opponents of compensation offer objections to it, and then its defenders respond. I am refusing to be led in this scholarly minuet by the opponents of donor compensation. To this end, I have argued in this chapter that the moral concern with securing donors' informed consent to donate requires that they be offered compensation.

To be clear, this conclusion is not that *all* plasma centers must offer their prospective donors compensation. So long as a system of uncompensated donation operated in the same area as a system of compensated donation the donors in the former system would have access to information concerning the level of compensation on offer for their plasma. If they needed this information to make an informed decision about whether or not to donate it would be available to them. Thus, to ensure that plasma collection agencies abide by the International Society of Blood Transfusion's Code of Ethics (that requires that "[t]he donor should provide informed consent to the donation of blood or blood components"), donor compensation must be allowed.[38]

Notes

1. Note that the superiority of these standards to the third – the "professional practice standard" – is assessed on grounds that are independent of the conclusion supported by the arguments in this volume.

2. See Chapter 1.
3. Tom L. Beauchamp and James F. Childress, *Principles of Biomedical Ethics* (New York: Oxford University Press, 2013, 7th edn), 120–121.
4. International Society of Blood Transfusion, "Code of Ethics, Clause 1," Available at: www.ncbi.nlm.nih.gov/pmc/articles/PMC4624526/#b3-blt-13-537. An argument for revising this code so that it is more patient-orientated has been provided by A. Farrugia and C. Del Bo, "Some Reflections on the Code of Ethics of the International Society of Blood Transfusion," *Blood Transfusion* 13, 4 (2015), 551–558. A response to Farrugia and Del Bo – albeit one marred by *ad hominem* attacks – is offered by Peter Flanagan, "The Code of Ethics of the International Society of Blood Transfusion," *Blood Transfusion* 13, 4 (2015), 537–538.
5. Beauchamp and Childress, *Principles of Biomedical Ethics*, 122.
6. The standard view is that the ethical requirement to secure a person's informed consent to the medical procedures that she is subject to is grounded on respect for her autonomy. It is important to note the caveat that autonomy is a foundational principle of Western bioethics; other cultural traditions might differ considerably here. See, for example, the discussion of the role of the family in medical decision-making in China in Mark J. Cherry and Ruiping Fan, "Informed Consent: The Decisional Standing of Families," *Journal of Medicine and Philosophy* 40 (2015), 363–370. Even in the West, the focus on the value of autonomy does not preclude there being space for family-based decision-making under certain conditions. This delegation could be understood in terms "of individual authority and autonomy," with persons being put on legal notice that under certain conditions (e.g., when their condition is "terminal or beset by an irreversible condition") the default position is that their family and/or physician will make decisions for them. Thus, if they do not object to this default arrangement it "is interpreted as implicitly authorized by the consent of the patient." See Mark J. Cherry and H. Tristram Engelhardt, Jr., "Informed Consent in Texas: Theory and Practice," *Journal of Medicine and Philosophy* 29, 2 (2004), 244.
7. An overview of the main analyses of personal autonomy can be found in James Stacey Taylor, "Introduction," *Personal Autonomy: New Essays on Personal Autonomy and Its Role in Contemporary Moral Philosophy* (Cambridge: Cambridge University Press, 2008), 1–31. Many accounts within the medical and regulatory literature hold that there are five elements involved in securing a person's informed consent: she must be competent to consent to the treatment in question, the information that is relevant to her decision must be disclosed to her, she must understand this information, she must make her decision voluntarily, and she must give her consent to her treatment. See, for example, Alan Meisel and Loren Roth, "What We Do and Do Not Know about Informed Consent," *Journal of the American Medical Association* 246 (1981), 2473–2477, and the National Commission for the Protection of Human Subjects of Biomedical and Behavioral Research, *The Belmont Report* (Washington, DC: DHEW Publication OS 78–0012, 1978), 10. Beauchamp and Childress expand this fivefold account of informed consent to a sevenfold account: the person must be competent "to understand and decide," act voluntarily in deciding, receive disclosure "of material information," receive a recommendation of a plan of action, and understand both the information and the plan presented to her; she must also decide in favor of a plan of action, and authorize that she be treated in accordance with it. Beauchamp and Childress, *Principles of Biomedical Ethics*, 125–140.

8. This agreement stems from the recognition that the Greek stems of "autonomy" are "autos" and "nomos" – "self" and "rule," respectively. See Edmund D. Pellegrino, "Patient and Physician Autonomy: Conflicting Rights and Obligations in the Physician-Patient Relationship," *Journal of Contemporary Health Law & Policy* 10, 1 (1994), 48. That autonomy is constituted by self-rule is agreed on by both Kantian and non-Kantian approaches to autonomy – although the analyses of this concept offered by the adherents of these different approaches to autonomy vary considerably. Kantian approaches holding that a person is autonomous to the extent that she is free from being guided by her desires and other pro-attitudes, while non-Kantian approaches – those that analyze autonomy as "personal" autonomy – hold that a person is autonomous to the degree that her effective first-order desires and her actions stem in some way from desires and values that are appropriately her own, and hence are those that she identifies with. For an account of the difference between these two approaches to autonomy see Harry G. Frankfurt, "Autonomy, Necessity, and Love," in Harry G. Frankfurt, ed., *Necessity, Volition, and Love* (Cambridge: Cambridge University Press, 1998), 134–136.
9. See James Stacey Taylor, "Autonomy and Informed Consent: A Much Misunderstood Relationship," *Journal of Value Inquiry* 38, 3 (2004), 383–391.
10. See Sheila A.M. McLean, *Autonomy, Consent, and the Law* (New York: Routledge-Cavendish, 2010), 42–46.
11. The legal view that the information that a person needed to be able to give her informed consent to her treatment should be measured by what a reasonable physician would disclose under the circumstances was established in *Nathanson v. Klein* 350 P2d (1093 Kan 1960).
12. See *Canturbury v. Spence* 464 F .2d 772 (D.C. Cir. 1972). This ruling replaced *Nathanson v. Klein*.
13. This claim is supported by a survey conducted of final year medical students that was conducted in the United Kingdom on the concept of medical professionalism that found that there was a "mix of values associated with different models of professionalism." Erica Borgstrom, Simon Cohn, and Stephen Barclay, "Medical Professionalism: Conflicting Values for Tomorrow's Doctors," *Journal of General Internal Medicine* 25, 12 (2010), 1330.
14. The possibility of such unethical behavior is supported by the data presented in Lisa I. Iezzoni, Sowmya R. Rao, Catherine M. DesRoches, Christine Vogeli, and Eric G. Campbell, "Survey Shows That At Least Some Physicians are not Always Open or Honest With Patients," *Health Affairs* 31, 2 (2012), 383–391.
15. McLean, *Autonomy, Consent, and the Law*, 83.
16. Beauchamp and Childress, *Principles of Biomedical Ethics*, 127.
17. That these two standards would converge on certain information being disclosed to patients follows from the view that this information would be needed by a reasonable patient combined with the default assumption (when applying the subjective standard) that each patient is a reasonable patient.
18. This is, as was discussed in Chapter 1, compatible with it being the case that offers of compensation – if sufficiently high – will lead to the donation of *more* blood and blood products than no compensation at all.
19. Carl Mellstrom and Magnus Johannesson, "Crowding Out in Blood Donation: Was Titmuss Right?" *Journal of the European Economic Association* 6, 4 (2008), 845–863.
20. Ibid., 849.
21. Ibid., 852.

22. Ibid.
23. Ibid., 857. They also note that "the potential problem of introducing monetary payments can be resolved by simply adding an option to donate the payment to charity."
24. Note that, despite the claims of some persons who oppose markets on moral grounds the fact that paying for a previously unpriced good will motivate some persons not to provide it does not undermine economic theory. For a version of this anti-market objection, see Michael J. Sandel, *What Money Can't Buy: The Moral Limits of Markets* (New York: Farrar, Straus and Giroux, 2012), 122. Instead, the phenomenon of crowding out is *predicted* by economic theory, for reasons that will become clear in the following.
25. For the sake of simplicity, the following discussion will focus on a person who ceases to donate once a certain level of compensation is offered to her.
26. This claim comes with a caveat; see note 27. A similar point is made in another context by Jeremy Shearmur, "The Gift Relationship Revisited," *HEC Forum* 27 (2015), 309.
27. This claim comes with a caveat: Assuming that the total amount of plasma secured when these donors were donating is that which needed to meet demand then such donors should cease to donate *provided* that their donations would be replaced by donations from donors whose opportunity costs were lower, such that (on this analysis) they should donate their plasma. And if the level of compensation that was being offered was an accurate reflection of the relationship between its supply and the demand for it this replacement would be expected to occur. (If it did not then the level of compensation would adjust accordingly, and then it would be the case that donors with higher opportunity costs should donate.) I thank an anonymous referee for pressing me on this point.
28. Although, again, see note 27.
29. Not all would-be donors would value their act of donation in this way; some would consider their act of donation to be beyond price, even when compensation is offered. But this argument in favor of the ethical necessity of offering compensation to the (typical) plasma donor does not rest on the claim that any actual donor would use the level of compensation that she is offered to ascribe value to her donation, but to the much weaker claim that it is plausible to hold that *some* would-be donors would do so.
30. Again, see note 27.
31. Securing a person's informed consent to donate will also require that she be informed if the organization to which she is considering donating will profit from her donation. Given that commercial plasma centers do not conceal their for-profit status, they will meet this condition. Some putatively non-profit centers, however, fail to reveal to donors that they will profit from the donations they receive (e.g., through selling recovered plasma to a commercial fractionator). They thus fail to secure the informed consent of (some of) their donors. See Brian Grainger and Peter Flanagan, "Informed Consent for Whole Blood Donation," *Vox Sanguinis* 115, 1 (2020), 6, and Patricia Mahon-Daly, "The Alienation of the Gift: The Ethical Use of Donated Blood," *Journal of Medical Law and Ethics* 3, 3 (2015), 200.
32. Recall that the professional practice standard of disclosure was rejected as the appropriate standard of disclosure earlier on grounds that were independent of the question of whether or not compensation should be offered to prospective plasma donors.
33. See Chapter 1.

34. Note that since a concern for informed consent requires that these donors be screened out in a system of plasma procurement that prohibits donor compensation, any current systems of plasma procurement that prohibit donor compensation and yet do *not* screen out this group of donors are undoubtedly securing plasma from persons who are unable to give their informed consent to donate. These systems are thus prima facie unethical.

35. That the Principle of Respect of Autonomy is one of the foundational principles of contemporary (Western) bioethics is widely recognized; see, for example, Beauchamp and Childress, *Principles of Biomedical Ethics*, Chapter 4, and R. Gillon, "Ethics Needs Principles – Four Can Encompass the Rest – and Respect for Autonomy Should be 'First Among Equals' " *Journal of Medical Ethics* 29 (2003), 307–312.

36. An argument for the view that the ethical requirement to secure a person's informed consent to her treatment rests on a moral concern with her well-being can be found in Taylor, "Autonomy and Informed Consent," 383–391. For an argument for the view that "informed consent is rooted in concerns about protecting and enabling autonomous or self-determining choice," see Ruth R. Faden, Tom L. Beauchamp, and Nancy M.P. King, *A History and Theory of Informed Consent* (New York: Oxford University Press, 1986), Chapter 7. (The quotation is from Faden et al., *A History and Theory of Informed Consent*, 235.) That the value of autonomy undergirds much of the Western concern with informed consent was noted by Shui Chuen Lee, "Intimacy and Family Consent: A Confucian Ideal," *Journal of Medicine and Philosophy* 40, 4 (2015), 419.

37. See, for example, McLean, *Autonomy, Consent, and the Law*, 69–97, and Alasdair Maclean, *Autonomy, Informed Consent, and Medical Law: A Relational Challenge* (New York: Cambridge University Press, 2009), Part II.

38. International Society of Blood Transfusion, "Code of Ethics, Clause 1."

3 Coercion, Force, Autonomy, and Consent

Introduction

In the previous chapter, I argued that the ethical requirement to secure a person's informed consent to any procedures that she is subject to requires that donor compensation be allowed. This ethical requirement of securing a person's informed consent is often justified by appeal to a moral concern for autonomy. A concern for donor autonomy (often glossed in the debate over donor compensation as donor "voluntariness") also underpins one of the most common objections to donor compensation: That if a person is motivated to donate by the offer of compensation then her autonomy with respect to her donation will be diminished as she will have thereby been coerced, or forced, into donating.[1]

Yet while this claim is widespread in discussions of compensated donation, little argument is ever offered for it. This is unfortunate, for it is possible to develop an argument for this position ("The Argument from Abdicated Control") that has considerable merit. But this possibility will provide only cold comfort for those who oppose compensating donors. This argument focuses on the question of whether presenting a person with an inducement could result in the diminution of her autonomy and concludes that it could. It thus supports their claim that inducements can (like threats) lead to a diminution in the autonomy of those who accept (or succumb to) them. But this conclusion leads to a problem: Since both threats and offers can function similarly to diminish the autonomy of those that succumb to (or accept) them, how can we distinguish between morally permissible and morally impermissible proposals?[2]

I argue in this chapter that the answer to this question can be drawn out of the concern that underlies the initial worry that certain offers (e.g., the offer of compensation to prospective plasma donors) would be coercive and hence impermissible. This concern is that in certain situations (e.g., those that involve coercion) a person's consent to a proposal (e.g., that made by her coercer) will be defective and, as such, will fail to authorize the transaction (or the proposer's treatment of her) to which she ostensibly agreed. Since in such cases the proposer will not have secured

DOI: 10.4324/9781003263913-4

authoritative consent from the person to whom she made the proposal, if she treats him as though she had secured his authoritative consent (and so consummates the interaction that she proposed) she will act wrongly. In the debate over donor compensation, the concern is that the consent of persons who donate their plasma for compensation will be defective owing to the background conditions (i.e., their economic impoverishment) against which they give it. If the consent of compensated donors is defective (and hence not authoritative), then plasma centers will act wrongly in accepting plasma from compensated donors.

The account of how a person's consent could be defective and hence not authoritative that I will provide in this chapter will be theoretically robust. But while it will capture the concerns of those who oppose compensating plasma donors on the (intuitive) grounds that they are coerced into donating, it will not support them. There is no reason to believe that compensated plasma donors will fail to meet the conditions for their consent to their donations to be authoritative (i.e., non-defective). But, I will argue, there is good reason to believe that when compensated donation is prohibited, the consent of persons who otherwise would have donated their plasma for compensation to refrain from so doing *would* be defective. Rather than plasma centers acting wrongly in offering compensation to prospective donors, then, those who *prohibit* such offers will act wrongly. The moral concern for donors that is expressed by those who oppose compensation on the grounds that it is somehow "coercive" should thus lead them to oppose the prohibition of donor compensation, not oppose its offer. Arguments from the putatively coercive nature of donor compensation thus backfire.

The Outline of This Chapter

The view that offers of compensation will compromise the autonomy of donors that accept them is both explicit and implicit in the literature on compensated donation. R.W. Beal and W.G. van Aken, for example, assert that the commercial procurement of blood carries with it a "risk" that the donors will be economically coerced into donating.[3] Similarly, Gilles Folléa, Erhard Seifried, and Jeroen de Wit write, "[a]s it may be more attractive to those from lower socio-economic groups who have a greater need to use this option to gain income, remuneration for blood could be viewed as coercion against donors, compromising their autonomous decision-making."[4] This view is also implicit in much of the discussion of the ethics of compensated donation. It is, for example, standard in the literature on compensated donation to refer to uncompensated donors as "voluntary non-remunerated donors" (VNRD) and their donations as "voluntary non-remunerated donations."[5] By contrast, compensated donors are routinely referred to merely as "remunerated donors" and their donations as "remunerated donations."[6] The implication is clear:

The donations of persons who do not receive financial compensation for donation are performed voluntarily while those of persons who have received compensation for their donation are not.

Yet despite the prevalence of the view that compensation renders a person's donation less than fully voluntary – that her autonomy with respect to it is somehow compromised – arguments for this position are either absent or underdeveloped.[7] This is unfortunate. Once it is expounded, this view has considerable merit. My first task in this chapter is thus to outline three ways in which this view could be supported. I will argue that two of the arguments that could be developed in its favor – the Argument from Economic Coercion and the Argument from Force – should be rejected. However, the third argument – the Argument from Abdicated Control – avoids the mistakes that are made by these arguments. Furthermore, this last argument captures the intuitive reason why it seems that procuring plasma through the offer of compensation is morally wrong – and does so in a way that avoids all of the standard responses that are offered by the defenders of donor compensation.

The Argument from Abdicated Control is both plausible and defensible. It supports the widely held (but rarely argued for) view that a person's autonomy with respect to her actions could be compromised by both threats and offers. But, as I noted earlier, this result leads to a problem: If both threats and offers could compromise a person's autonomy with respect to the actions that she performs in response to them, how can morally permissible proposals be distinguished from morally impermissible proposals? I argue that the standard focus on determining whether a particular proposal is a "threat" or an "offer" (or, possibly, a "coercive offer") as a way of determining whether or not it is morally permissible is mistaken.[8] Instead, the moral permissibility or otherwise of the consummation of a particular proposal should be assessed against the question of whether the person who acceded to it consented to it a way that ensures that her consent is authoritative.

In providing a theoretically satisfying account of how successfully subjecting a person to coercion compromises her autonomy with respect to the acts that she is coerced into performing the Argument from Abdicated Control thus shifts the debate from one focused on donor autonomy to one focused on donor consent. With this recognition in hand, I will develop an account of the conditions that must be met for a person's consent to be authoritative. I will then argue that there is reason to believe that compensated donors will give their authoritative consent to donate for compensation. It is thus permissible for plasma centers to offer compensation to their prospective donors and exchange this for their donations. But, I will argue, when donor compensation is prohibited, many prospective plasma donors will *not* give their authoritative consent to be precluded from receiving compensation for their donations. The prohibition of donor compensation is thus impermissible. A moral concern for donor "voluntariness" thus supports allowing donor compensation and opposes its prohibition.

The Argument From Coercion

An initial argument in support of the view that the offer of compensation would compromise the autonomy of those who accept it could be dubbed the "Argument from Economic Coercion." This argument begins with the empirical claim that many prospective plasma donors who would be induced to donate by the offer of cash compensation would be relatively poor.[9] They thus need the compensation that is offered for their plasma not to improve their situation but only to prevent it from becoming worse.[10] The argument then continues with the normative claim that personal autonomy is of considerable moral value. It then holds that, since this is so, social institutions that promote its development and protect it once it is developed are morally preferable to those that do not. The argument then claims that successfully subjecting persons to coercion will compromise their autonomy with respect to the actions that they are coerced into performing. Drawing on its initial empirical claim its proponents then infer that those donors who are motivated to donate by the offer of financial compensation are coerced into so doing by their economic situation. Since successfully subjecting persons to coercion will compromise their autonomy, and since social institutions that promote the development of personal autonomy and protect it once it is developed are morally preferable to those that do not, social institutions that protect persons from being coerced by their economic situation into performing certain actions (e.g., plasma donation) would be morally preferable to those that do not. Prohibiting plasma centers from offering financial compensation to prospective donors would prevent the donors' economic situation from coercing them into donating to secure the preferred compensation. Thus, since social institutions that prevent this would be morally preferable to those that would not, it would be morally preferable to prohibit donor compensation rather than to permit it. Thus, the proponents of this argument conclude, donor compensation should, morally, be prohibited.

The primary aim of this Argument from Coercion is to establish that offering financial compensation to plasma donors is morally wrong. But it can also provide an explanation of why there is (putatively) a moral difference between plasma centers offering to compensate prospective donors with cash and offering to compensate them with noncash benefits, such as lottery tickets or paid days off work.[11] The proponents of this argument hold that many persons who would be motivated to donate their plasma by the offer of cash compensation would do so because they need it. However, while such prospective donors would need cash, they would not need lottery tickets or paid days off work. Thus, if they donated plasma to secure these goods, they would do so because they freely chose to pursue them, not because they had to pursue them to survive. They would thus not be coerced by their economic situation into donating but would be fully autonomous with respect to their donations.[12]

The Argument from Coercion is mistaken. I grant that the proponents of this argument are correct to note that successfully subjecting a person to coercion will compromise her autonomy with respect to the actions that she is coerced into performing.[13] I also grant for the sake of argument that they are correct that some persons only donate to receive the offered compensation solely to prevent their situation from becoming worse. With respect to the reasons for which they were performed, these acts will resemble acts that a person is motivated to perform through coercion. But there are important differences between the acts performed by a person who is coerced into performing them and the act of donation performed by a financially desperate donor. (Again, note that I have granted that such donors exist for the sake of argument.) These differences undermine this argument.

Coercion and Autonomy

To assess the Argument from Coercion, it is necessary to establish how successfully subjecting a person to coercion will compromise her autonomy with respect to the acts that she is coerced into performing. This is not as simple as it might at first appear. One cannot appeal to a hierarchical analysis of autonomy (on which, roughly, a person will be autonomous with respect to the action that she performs if she wants to perform the action, and also wants to want to perform this action and wants her first-order desire to perform it to be effective in leading her to act) to claim that a person who is coerced into performing an action does not do what she really wants to do.[14] Although there is a sense in which a person who is coerced into performing an action does not do what she really wants to do (just as there is a sense in which a person who donates her plasma only out of economic necessity does not do what she really wants to do), there is a more important sense in which she *does* do what she really wants to do. A person who is coerced into performing an action will have decided that, given the threat that she is faced with, the action that her coercer desires her to perform to avoid the penalty that he is threatening her with is that which she desires to perform in this situation.[15] Moreover, a person who is successfully coerced into performing an action will desire that she desires to perform the action that she is being coerced into performing and will desire that her first-order desire to perform it will lead her to act. Any countervailing desire that she might experience to act differently (such as to resist) would be one that she would wish to quash for fear of the threatened consequences of non-compliance with her coercer's demands. There is a sense, then, in which a person who is successfully coerced into performing an action *does* do what she really wants to do. It thus seems that on a standard hierarchical account of autonomy successfully subjecting a person to coercion will not compromise her autonomy.

This conclusion will strike many as absurd – and with good reason. Imagine someone who is constantly followed around by a person who always holds a loaded gun to his head and who has informed him that she will kill him if he performs any action other than those that she tells him to perform. Such a person would not be a paradigm of autonomy, of self-direction, even though he only performed actions that, given the circumstances that he was in, he really wanted to perform.

An analysis of how successfully coercing a person into performing a particular action will compromise her autonomy with respect to that action must thus accommodate two apparently conflicting intuitions. First, it must accommodate the intuition that a person who is coerced into performing an action performs the action that, given the circumstances that she is in, she really wants to perform. (This intuition supports the view that coercing a person into performing an action will not compromise her autonomy.) Second, it must accommodate the intuition that a person who is coerced into performing an action will lack self-direction with respect to it; that it will not be she, but her coercer, who is directing her performance of it. (This intuition supports the view that coercing a person into performing an action will compromise her autonomy.)

These apparently conflicting intuitions can be accommodated once it is recognized both that autonomy is a property of persons with respect both to their decisions and their actions, and that a person is autonomous with respect to her decisions or her actions if it is she, and not someone else, who exercises control over (respectively) their content and nature (i.e., what actions she performs).[16] More precisely, a person will be autonomous with respect to her decisions if she meets three conditions with respect to them. The first of these is

> The Threshold Condition: For a person to be autonomous with respect to a decision that she makes it is necessary that (i) the information on which she based the decision has not been affected by another agent ("the manipulative agent") with the end of leading her to make a particular decision, or a decision from a particular class of decisions; or (ii) if the information on which a person bases her decision has been affected by a manipulative agent then she is aware of the way in which it has been so affected; and (iii) if the information on which a person bases her decision has been affected by a manipulative agent and if she is not aware of the way in which the information on which she is basing her decision has been so affected, then she did not make the decision that the manipulative agent intended her to make.[17]

The Threshold Condition outlines the conditions that are necessary for a person to be autonomous with respect to her decisions. But it does not provide sufficient conditions for this. (A young child, for example, could meet the Threshold Condition with respect to some of her decisions, but she would not be autonomous with respect to them.) This condition thus needs to be supplemented with

> The Degree Condition: (i) The maximum degree to which a person will be autonomous with respect to a decision that she makes will be determined by the degree to which it is the result of a decision-making procedure that she is satisfied with (i.e., she believes she has sufficient reason to continue using it) as being her decision-making procedure for making the type of decision that is in question; to the degree that the genesis of her decision departs from this her autonomy with respect to the decision in question will be diminished, and (ii) the person's satisfaction with her decision-making procedure will meet The Threshold Condition.[18]

As stated, the Degree Condition is static and so would preclude a person from being autonomous with respect to a new type of decision-making procedure that she had (autonomously) decided to try out with respect to certain types of decisions. To avoid this, these initial two conditions need to be supplemented with a third:

> Tracking Condition: If a person decides to use a different decision-making procedure than that which she is satisfied with as being her own, then the maximal degree to which she is autonomous with respect to the decisions that she makes using it will be determined by the degree to which she is autonomous with respect to the decision-making procedure that she (i) used to make the choice to use an alternative decision-making procedure, and (ii) used to make the choice to use the particular alternative decision-making procedure that she uses. Her degree of autonomy with respect to the decisions that she makes will then be determined by how closely her actual decision-making procedure that leads to them is in accord with the decision-making procedure that she decided to adopt in making them.[19]

A person who has been coerced into performing a particular action could still be fully autonomous with respect to her decision to perform it. She would have been aware of the way in which the information on which she based her decision had been affected by her coercer (who would be "the manipulative agent" in this case) and so she would satisfy the Threshold Condition. Her decision to submit to his demands could have been arrived at through a decision-making procedure that she was satisfied with, where her satisfaction with this procedure met the Threshold

Condition. She can also be fully autonomous with respect to her decision to comply by meeting the Tracking Condition: If she used a different decision-making procedure than that which she was satisfied with as being her own then she could still be fully autonomous with respect to her decision to use it in this instance.

That a person who is coerced into performing a particular action could be fully autonomous with respect to her decision to perform it captures the intuition that she does what she really wants to do. However, that she is fully autonomous with respect to her decision to perform the action that her coercer instructs her to perform does not entail that she is thereby fully autonomous with respect to her performance of that action. This is because it is not she *but her coercer* who decides which action she is to perform. She merely decides to perform whatever action he requires of her to avoid the penalty that he threatens her with.[20] In making this decision and then acting upon it (i.e., by performing the action that her coercer instructs her to perform), she abdicates control over the actions that she performs to her coercer. To the extent that this is so her autonomy with respect to the actions that she thus performs at his behest will be compromised. This captures the intuition that a person who is coerced into performing an action will lack self-direction with respect to it; that it will not be she, but her coercer, who is directing her performance of it.

The Argument From Coercion Fails

A person who is successfully coerced into performing a particular action will thus have her autonomy with respect to that action compromised to the extent that she has abdicated control over her actions to her coercer, and so it is accordingly he, and not she, who controls her performance of the action in question. For a person to have her autonomy compromised through being subject to coercion she must be coerced *by an agent* to whom she can abdicate control over her actions. It is this abdication of control that results in the compromise of her autonomy. But this entails that *non*-agential forces (such as her economic situation) cannot coerce her into performing particular actions (such as donating plasma for compensation). The Argument from Coercion thus fails because its central claim – that donors who are motivated to donate by the offer of cash compensation are coerced into so doing by their economic situation – is false.

The Argument From Force

The proponents of the Argument from Coercion have a response to the earlier criticism.[21] This is that to construe their objection to allowing compensation to be offered to prospective donors of plasma as one that is solely concerned with protecting persons from *coercion* is to construe it too narrowly. Their real concern is not that (the typical) prospective donors of plasma would (properly speaking) be *coerced* by their economic situation into donating if compensation were offered. Instead, their concern is whether they would, given their situation, see themselves as having *no other viable choice* but to donate – whether they would see themselves as being *forced* into donating.[22] And, the proponents of this "Argument from Force" could continue, if a person is forced into donating in this way, then her actions will be dictated to her by her situation. To the extent that this is so, then, she will lack self-direction, autonomy, with respect to the acts that she is forced into performing. Hence, a concern for the value of autonomy would require that persons be protected from situations in which they see themselves as having only one viable course of action available to them. And, the proponents of this argument continue, some prospective donors of plasma would believe that their only viable option to secure the money that they needed was to donate. Since this is so removing this option from their choice set would protect them from being in a situation in which they believed that they only had one viable course of action available to them. Hence, the proponents of this argument conclude compensation for plasma donation should be prohibited to protect donor autonomy.

As it is outlined here, the Argument from Force is incomplete in two respects. The first of these lacunae arises from the obvious oddity of this line of argument: Its proponents are consciously proposing to remove from the choice set of the impoverished prospective donors of plasma the option that these donors consider to be the best one available to them.[23] To justify prohibiting offers of compensation to prospective plasma donors, the proponent of the Argument from Force must thus establish that the value of preventing the autonomy of prospective donors from being compromised as a result of their being forced in this way to donate their plasma is *objectively greater* than the value of the benefits that they would receive from receiving compensation for donating. The second of these lacunae is that for this argument to be complete its proponents must establish that plasma donors are forced into donating in the way that this argument claims.

The Argument From Force and the Objective Value of Autonomy

There are two lines of argument that the proponent of the Argument from Force could offer to establish that the value of preventing the autonomy of prospective donors from being compromised as a result of their being forced in this way to donate their plasma is *objectively greater* than the value of the benefits that they would receive from receiving compensation for donating. She could argue that autonomy is of such great value that no amount of increase in a person's well-being could justify any compromise of her autonomy. Alternatively, she could argue that the compensation that a desperate donor would receive for her plasma would be inadequate to compensate her for her plasma, her time, and the degree to which her autonomy was compromised. The first line of argument is grounded on the value of autonomy and will be addressed shortly. The second line of argument, however, is not primarily concerned with protecting donor autonomy. Instead, it is primarily concerned with the claim that donors will not receive a just price for what they give up in donating. I will address this claim – that donors will be *exploited* by those plasma centers that offer them compensation – in the next two chapters.

It is commonplace to hold that personal autonomy is of great value.[24] But it is not. Consider Othello in Shakespeare's play of that name.[25] Othello was manipulated by Iago into making the decisions (and consequently performing the acts) that Iago wanted him to perform. Since Othello was unaware of Iago's machinations, he was not autonomous with respect to the decisions that Iago manipulated him into making. He failed to meet either criterion (i) of the Threshold Condition ("the information on which she based the decision has not been affected by another agent . . . with the end of leading her to make a particular decision, or a decision from a particular class of decisions") or criterion (ii) ("if the information on which a person bases her decision has been affected by a manipulative agent then she is aware of the way in which it has been so affected"). Now consider a variant on *Othello* (*McOthello*) in which all the characters are honest Scotsmen. Instead of providing information to McOthello with the aim of manipulating him into making certain decisions, McIago merely provides him with what he, McIago, believes to be true information. Alas, this is precisely the same information that Iago provided to Othello in the original version of the play, and precisely the same events transpire. However, since McIago is not manipulating McOthello, McOthello satisfies the Threshold Condition (and also, *ex hypothesi*, the Degree Condition and the Trading Condition). Unlike Othello, then, McOthello is fully autonomous with respect to both his decisions and the actions that flow from them. But since precisely the same actions and events occur in both *Othello* and *McOthello*, both situations should be valued identically – even though McOthello was far more autonomous with respect to his actions than was Othello. McOthello's autonomy thus had no value in itself.[26] There is thus no reason to believe that autonomy is of such great value that no amount of increase in a person's well-being could justify any diminution in her autonomy.[27] The first line of argument that the defender of the Argument from Force could offer to show that the value of preventing the autonomy of prospective donors from being compromised is necessarily objectively greater than that of the benefits that they would receive from being compensated for their donation fails.

But perhaps this response to the first line of argument that a defender of the Argument from Force could offer moves too quickly. The claim that the situations in *Othello* and *McOthello* should be valued identically could be challenged in two ways. First, one might hold that the situation in *McOthello* is morally preferable to that of *Othello* (and hence is more valuable) since McIago lacked the malice of Iago. Second, one might hold that if Othello and McOthello had interests in exercising their autonomy then, again, the situation in *McOthello* should be valued higher than that of *Othello* because (assuming that the interest-based account of well-being is correct) McOthello would possess a higher degree of well-being than Othello. Both of these challenges are contentious. It is not obvious that the bare wrong of having a malicious mental state would render a situation in which this was true morally worse than one where it was not, and the interest-based account of well-being has faced trenchant criticism from hedonists.[28] But even if these two challenges are sound (and so the situations in *Othello* and *McOthello* should be valued differently), they do not undermine the earlier response to the Argument from Force. This is because, first, the (putative) differences in the moral preferability or the value of these situations are not grounded on claims concerning the *autonomy* (or lack thereof) of McOthello and Othello. The claim that the situation in *McOthello* is morally preferable to that of *Othello* because McIago lacked the malicious mental states of Iago is based on an assessment of these situations' moral worth, not on an assessment of the value of the autonomy that is held or lacked within them. Similarly, even if it is accepted that McOthello is better off than Othello as his interest in autonomy is fulfilled, the difference in value between his situation and that of Othello is grounded on the value of well-being, not on the value of autonomy. The example of *Othello* and *McOthello* thus shows that there is no reason to believe that autonomy has any value in itself.

The Argument From Force and Donor Autonomy

This initial discussion of the Argument from Force has proceeded on the assumption that a person who donated plasma to receive the offered compensation would have had her autonomy with respect to her act of donation compromised as a result of being forced to donate by her economic desperation. As I noted earlier, this assumption must be justified by the proponent of this argument. Unfortunately for the proponents of this argument, they will be unable to justify this assumption as it is unwarranted. Not only is there no reason to believe that any actual donors are forced in this way to donate, there is reason to believe that they are *not* forced into donating. Their autonomy with respect to their acts of donation is thus not compromised at all.

To establish that donors are forced into donating by the economic desperation, the proponents of the Argument from Force must provide an account of what it means for a person to be "forced" into donating such that her autonomy with respect to her act of donating is compromised. Then, with this account in hand, they must show that actual donors are forced into donating.

The proponents of the Argument from Force hold that a donor who donates out of desperation to secure the compensation offered to her will thereby be forced into donating and hence her autonomy with respect to her act of donation will be diminished. As with the Argument from Coercion, this argument is based on the claim that it is the donors' economic situation that, in conjunction with the offer of compensation for their plasma, leads to their autonomy with respect to their act of donating being compromised. It is not based on the claim that desperate donors suffer from a diminution in their autonomy as a result of being subjected to the will of another agent. The proponents of this argument must thus accept that the (putatively) desperate donors that they are concerned with meet the Threshold Condition for being autonomous with respect to their act of donation. Moreover, since there is no reason to believe that these donors are systematically unsatisfied with their decision-making procedures (as opposed to being systematically unsatisfied with the options that they are faced with), they should also accept that these donors could meet both the Degree Condition and the Tracing Condition. This being so, the only way in which the proponents of this argument could continue to hold that the desperate donors that they are concerned with would suffer from a diminution in their autonomy with respect to their donations *is to deny that they are deciding to act at all* when faced with the offer of compensation. The sense of "force" that this argument rests on thus must be that on which a person's movements do not stem from her own agency but from a non-agential force that is external to her. On this view, then, a person who is forced to donate by the offer of compensation would be like someone who is forced over a waterfall by a swiftly rushing river that has carried her away. In neither case were the persons concerned (the donor, the victim of the waterfall) autonomous with respect to the overall motions of their bodies for in neither case were these motions the result of decisions or actions for which the question of her autonomy could arise.

When outlined this starkly, it is evident that the Argument from Force is unsound. It is absurd to think that even the most economically desperate of plasma donors ceases to act and is simply reduced to the level of an automaton when faced with an offer of compensation.[29] Yet before moving to consider an alternative (and far more plausible) autonomy-based objection to donor compensation it must be acknowledged that the Argument from Force captures an intuition about autonomy that underlies some analyses of this concept that differ from that outlined earlier. The intuitive appeal of the claim that a donor who is motivated to donate by the offer of compensation is forced into donating is based on the view that such donors will have such limited options that which they consider to be the best available to them is still unpalatable. Their situation thus forces them into choosing that option (e.g., to donate plasma). As such, *they* are not directing their actions, *their situation* is, and so to the extent that this is so they lack autonomy.

But while this view is widespread it is erroneous. It conflates a person's being autonomous with her autonomy being of instrumental value to her. Consider a situation in which a man is trapped in a pit.[30] His friends are unable to rescue him, but they can lower food to him each day. Being poor, they eat either fish or vegetables each day, and they give the man in the pit the same choice of which to eat. Neither this man's decisions nor his actions are subject to the will of another. He is thus fully autonomous, fully self-directed, with respect to them. But given his situation his autonomy is of little value to him for the options that he has available are so limited. Similarly, from the point of view of one who values autonomy highly the problem with the situation of the economically desperate donors is not that they lack autonomy, but that given their limited choices their autonomy is of little value to them. But the correct response to this state of affairs is not to make it even less valuable to them by making their pursuit of what they take to be their best option (e.g., the donation of plasma) more costly to them by imposing penalties (e.g., by prohibiting compensation) on them if they pursue it. If the Argument from Force is marshalled to oppose compensated plasma donation it will thus backfire.

The Argument From Abdicated Control

Both the Argument from Coercion and the Argument from Force fail because they are based on the mistaken view that a person's autonomy with respect to her decisions and actions can be compromised solely by her being in a situation in which she has few viable options. The proponents of the Argument from Abdicated Control do not make this mistake.[31] They accept that a person's autonomy with respect to her decisions and her actions can only be compromised when another agent usurps control over these. They also accept the objection that was offered against the Argument from Coercion – that a person's autonomy with respect to the actions that she is coerced into performing is only compromised as a result of her deciding to cede control over them to her coercer. But they note that offering compensation to a person to induce her to donate her plasma could have the same effect on her autonomy as threatening her with a penalty if she does not consent to donate. A person who is successfully coerced by another into donating her plasma would have decided to "Perform any action that my coercer requires of me from within that set of actions that I would rather perform that receive the threatened penalty."[32] She thus decides to cede control over her actions to her coercer.

To the extent that this is so her autonomy with respect to those actions would be compromised. (This example is offered for illustrative purposes only. I do not mean to imply that any actual plasma donor is coerced in this way.) But a person who is induced to donate her plasma by the offer of compensation would similarly have her autonomy compromised with respect to her act of donation. To receive the compensation on offer she would have decided to "Perform any action that my enticer requires of me from within that set of actions that I would be willing to perform to receive the offered compensation." As with the coerced donor, the induced donor would also have decided to cede control over her actions to the person who was offering her compensation for her plasma. To the extent that this was so her autonomy with respect to her act of donation would be compromised. Hence, the proponent of the Argument from Abdicated Control concludes, since both coercion and inducement can have the same effects on the autonomy of donors with respect to their acts of donation offering compensation to prospective donors of plasma can be functionally equivalent to coercion. Thus, if a concern for the value of personal autonomy should lead one *prima facie* to oppose subjecting persons to coercion, it should also lead one *prima facie* to oppose allowing plasma centers to offer donor compensation.[33]

Two-Tier Consent

A defender of donor compensation might object that the Argument from Abdicated Control should be rejected as it proves too much. The conclusion of this argument is not merely that plasma donors will have their autonomy compromised with respect to their acts of donation. It is the far broader conclusion that *anyone* who accepts an offer to perform an action specified in part by the person making the offer will have her autonomy compromised with respect to the actions that she performs at his behest. Thus, if one believes that acts that would adversely affect the autonomy of another are *prima facie* impermissible then one should *prima facie* oppose all offers. But this is absurd. So, the Argument from Abdicated Control should be rejected.

But while this response is initially persuasive it moves too quickly. It correctly notes that the earlier argument establishes that offers have the same effect on the autonomy of those who accept them as threats have on the autonomy of those who succumb to them. It then concludes that since it would be absurd to hold that all offers are thereby impermissible the argument should be rejected. But the conclusion of the Argument from Abdicated Control is not that it is morally impermissible *simpliciter* for plasma centers to offer compensation to prospective donors. It is the conditional claim that *if* a concern for the value of personal autonomy should lead one *prima facie* to oppose subjecting persons to coercion, *then* it should also lead one *prima facie* to oppose allowing plasma centers to offer donor compensation. Rather than rejecting this Argument *in toto*, one could instead accept its analysis of the effects that threats and offers have on the autonomy of those who succumb to them or accept them, but deny the antecedent of its conditional conclusion. That is, one could accept that a person who accepts an offer and as a result acts at the behest of another has her autonomy with respect to the acts that she thus performs compromised but deny that this renders the offer impermissible.

But if a concern for the value of personal autonomy cannot help us to distinguish between the proposals that are morally permissible (e.g., uncoercive offers) from those that are not (e.g., coercive offers and threats), what can? Before turning to answer this, I should emphasize that the question at hand is *not* the conceptual question of how threats can be distinguished from offers. Nor is it the conceptual question of whether or not offers can be coercive. Instead, it is the *normative* question of what conditions must be met for a proposal to be morally permissible. The reason for this is simple. The focus on the conceptual questions of whether threats can be distinguished from offers (and, if not, whether offers can be coercive) is often motivated by two related beliefs. The first belief is that while successfully threatening a person would compromise her autonomy motivating her to behave in a certain way through successfully making an offer to her would not. Thus, while threats are impermissible offers are not. The second belief is that if an offer could be shown to be coercive (i.e., it is a "coercive offer") then, since it could thus adversely affect the autonomy of the person to whom it was presented, it would be *prima facie* wrongful. However, in outlining the Argument from Abdicated Control, I argued that threats and offers can function equivalently with respect to their effects on the autonomy of those who (respectively) comply with them or accept them. From the point of view of one concerned with the moral value of autonomy, the permissibility or otherwise of a proposal thus cannot be determined by categorizing it as a "threat" (impermissible) or an offer (permissible) or even as a "coercive offer" (impermissible).[34] The question is thus not how to categorize a proposal (e.g., the proposal to provide compensation for plasma) as a threat or an offer but how to distinguish between proposals whose proffering and consequent consummation are morally permissible from those whose proffering and consequent consummation are not.[35]

Since concern for the value of autonomy cannot distinguish between those proposals whose offer and consummation are morally permissible and those that are not, what can? As I indicated earlier in this chapter, the answer lies with whether the consent of the person to whom the proposal is made is authoritative or not. But securing a person's authoritative consent to her treatment is not valuable for its own sake. It is valuable as this is likely to protect or promote her well-being. This approach is supported by the initially plausible claim that a proposal that a person accepts as she believes that it will make her better off is morally permissible while a proposal that she accepts only to prevent her situation from becoming worse is morally impermissible. In the former case, it is plausible to claim that since she expects her consent to advance her interests beyond the baseline of her current situation it is authoritative, while in the latter case she would merely be trying to retain her current baseline of well-being. She would have thus been in some sense pressured into consenting by her situation, and so her consent is not authoritative but defective.

But while this initial attempt to distinguish between those proposals whose offer and consummation are permissible and those where this combination is impermissible is plausible it is false. It would not be morally permissible for a woman to offer (and then provide) professional advancement to a man in return for sexual favors unrelated to his job even if he accepts as he considers this offer to be, on balance, one that would make him better off. (He knows that she would not retaliate in any way if he were to decline this offer, so he would not accept it to prevent his situation from getting worse.) And it would not be morally impermissible for a person to offer and then to sell a pill to someone in the initial stages of a naturally occurring debilitating disease (and to whom she owed no independent duty to provide this) even though she knows that he would buy it only to prevent his situation from becoming worse.

Yet the falsity of this initially plausible claim does not undercut the plausibility of the view that morally permissible proposals are to be distinguished from morally impermissible proposals by reference to their respective effects on the well-being of the persons to whom they are made. But capturing the plausibility of this view is complicated by the fact (noted earlier) that in cases of both morally permissible (e.g., a lucrative offer of morally permissible employment) and morally impermissible (e.g., "Your money or your life!") proposals the person to whom the proposal is made really wanted to accept it, given the situation that she was in. There is thus in both cases a sense in which she was made better off by accepting both types of proposal. But this sense comes with a caveat – *given the situation that she was in* she was made better off by accepting the proposal. The situation in which a proposal is made to a person is thus relevant to its moral permissibility. But it would be mistaken to attempt to distinguish between proposals whose offer and consummation are permissible and those where this combination is impermissible by identifying the latter as those that would be accepted in a situation that the person to whom it was made would prefer not to be in while the former would be accepted in one with which she was satisfied. A person who accepts and consummates a (morally permissible) proposal thereby indicates that she would prefer to be in a situation different from that which she was in prior to the proposal being made and consummated (i.e., she would prefer to be in the situation she anticipates being in after accepting the proposal). Similarly, certain conditional offers of aid to persons in desperate situations who then receive the aid in question after agreeing to its terms are morally permissible even though the person to whom these offers are made would prefer to be situated differently (i.e., in a situation where they did not require aid).

But while this discussion has not (yet) provided an account of how to distinguish proposals whose offer and consummation are morally permissible from those for whom this is not the case it has yielded two data points: That a promising way to distinguish between permissible and impermissible proposal-and-consummation pairs will rest on their effects on the recipient's well-being, and that the situation of the person to whom they are made is relevant to assessing their permissibility. This second point serves as a constraint on the first. Given the situation that they were in, persons would be willing to accept (i.e., consummate) intuitively impermissible proposals as they would think that this would be the best way to secure their well-being. Thus, the mere fact that a person would be made better off by accepting a proposal when compared to the situation where she did not accept it will not render the combination of its proffering and consequent consummation morally permissible.

An account of how to distinguish morally permissible from impermissible proposal and consummation pairs thus cannot focus only on whether the person to whom a proposal was made would accept it out of concern for her own well-being. It must also focus on whether her concern for her well-being would lead her to desire that the *type* of proposal that she received be generally allowed (and accepted) or generally precluded. This additional requirement will capture the idea that certain exchanges that a person might wish to consummate *given her situation* (e.g., her money for her life when faced with a highwayman) might still result from proposals (e.g., "Your money or your life!") whose consummation would be morally impermissible. Consider again the man who was offered professional advancement in exchange for sexual favors. He might be willing to accept this offer as it would make him better off. But, given his subaltern status as a male in a female-dominated professional environment, he might prefer that such offers not be allowed. He might think that were such offers disallowed his career would be the same as it would have been had they been allowed (i.e., had he accepted the inappropriate offer of his female supervisor) but he would not have had to perform sexual favors to achieve this.

Thus, for a proposal and its consequent consummation to be morally permissible two conditions must be met: (1) Given the situation that they are in both parties would be autonomous with respect to their preference that the proposed token exchange take place rather than not and (2) both parties would be autonomous with respect to their preference that exchanges of *that type* are allowed rather than precluded as both believe that allowing them could lead to an increase in their respective well-being.[36]

Two-Tier Consent and the Narrowing Bounds of Permissible Exchange

From the earlier discussion, it is clear that condition (1) will be met even by proposed exchanges that are morally impermissible (e.g., those made by highwaymen). So, the real test is whether or not (2) will be met. This might not appear to be an especially novel requirement. But this appearance is deceptive: This requirement has some striking implications. First, it represents a significant move away from the standard defense that is often offered to establish that certain proposed exchanges are morally permissible.[37] Like the account outlined earlier, the standard defense of the permissibility of exchange appeals to the value of well-being. It holds that if persons would voluntarily exchange certain goods and services if markets in them were permitted this provides a *prima facie* justification for allowing such markets, as persons would not engage in transactions unless they believed that they would make them better off. This is widely regarded as a plausible *prima facie* justification of markets. But with the earlier discussion in hand, this defense can now be seen merely to be a version of condition (1). And as I noted earlier (e.g., in the context of the sexually harassing offer) this alone cannot distinguish those proposed exchanges whose consummation is morally permissible from those that are not.[38]

Second, requiring that (2) be met by a proposed exchange for its offer and consequent consummation to be morally permissible shows that certain exchanges that persons might be willing to engage in voluntarily are still impermissible. Consider markets in votes. James Tobin wrote that "Any good second year graduate student in economics could write a short examination paper proving that voluntary transactions in votes would increase the welfare of the sellers as well as the buyers" – a claim that has been drawn upon by Christopher Freiman to defend vote markets.[39] But while allowing a market in votes could increase the welfare of both buyers and sellers given the situation that they are in (i.e., one in which a market in votes is permitted), this does not show that they would prefer that a market in votes be allowed. Consider a hypothetical situation in which there are 100 voters, of whom 10 are rich and 90 are poor, and two Parties, the Rich Party and the Poor Party. The Rich Party is far better capitalized than the Poor Party. All voters are rationally self-interested, vote solely in their economic self-interest, and only value their votes as instruments to change the outcome of elections. Absent a market in votes either the Poor Party would invariably win (if both Parties have policies that would advance the interests of their natural constituents to the serious financial detriment of persons in the other financial class) or both Parties would adjust their policies to appeal to the median voter.[40] However, if a market in votes was to be allowed not only would the Rich

Party invariably win but it could do so even if it had policies that would favor the Rich to the financial detriment of the Poor. No individual vote is likely to be pivotal in any given election. There is thus no reason for any individual voter to refuse to sell her vote to the highest bidder for it does not matter to the outcome of the election whether she does so or not. Each Poor voter would thus be motivated to sell her vote to the Rich Party. But the Rich Party does not need to purchase all of the Poor votes to ensure electoral success; it only needs 51 of them. (This would guarantee success even if no Rich voter voted.) Recognizing this, the Poor voters would compete to sell their votes to the Rich Party. Since votes are fungible, the Poor voters could only compete on price. The price of a vote would thus fall to just above transaction costs. Both the Poor voters who sold their votes and those who did not would suffer from financial loss as a result of the ensuring Rich Party victory. To establish that exchanges of votes for cash would enhance the well-being of both parties to them one should thus not ask whether these parties *would participate in these exchanges* if they were allowed. Instead, one should ask whether both parties to the proposed exchange *would want these exchanges to be allowed.* That condition (1) is met thus does not establish that an exchange is *prima facie* morally permissible on the basis of a moral concern for the well-being of those who would participate in it; condition (2) must also be met.[41] And since some exchanges that are favored by market advocates will fail to meet condition (2), it is a more stringent requirement than it might at first appear.

Back to Donor Compensation

The proposal of financial compensation for plasma and the consequent exchange of cash for plasma donation could meet both conditions (1) and (2). (Such exchanges stem from what could be termed "activation proposals" as they are attempts to initiate the activation of a positive exchange of goods or services.) Given the situations that they are in both the persons operating the plasma center and prospective donors could decide that they would rather engage in the proposed exchange of plasma for compensation than not. (And they would both so decide if any such actual exchange took place.) Assuming that the persons involved are autonomous with respect to these decisions, this proposed exchange would thus meet condition (1). It could also meet condition (2). Both the persons operating the plasma center and prospective donors could autonomously decide that they would rather have exchanges of that type be allowed rather than precluded on the grounds that they both believe that allowing them could lead to an increase in their respective well-being. The offer of financial compensation for plasma and the consequent consummation of plasma donation for financial compensation are thus likely to be morally permissible. The concern that plasma donors' consent to their donations would be defective owing to the background conditions against which they consented is thus misplaced.

But things are different when we turn to consider the moral permissibility of *prohibiting* plasma centers from compensating donors. An attempt to *prevent* an exchange (e.g., of plasma for cash) can be construed as a proposed exchange (a "prohibitive proposal") in the same way that the highwayman's demand of "Your money or your life!' could be construed as an exchange. That is, it could be understood as a proposal to refrain from performing an action (i.e., the imposition of penalties) in exchange for *either* the performance of a specified action (e.g., handing over one's wallet) *or* refraining from performing a specified action (e.g., not exchanging compensation for plasma) on the part of the person (or persons) to whom the offer was made. And, like the highwayman's demand, the prohibition of compensated donation could fail to satisfy both of the conditions that must be met for its related proposal and consummation pair to be morally permissible. Like the highwayman and her victim, both of the parties to the proposed exchange (i.e., a refraining from the imposition of penalties in exchange for the refraining from donating plasma for compensation) could satisfy condition (1). Given the situation that they are in, the persons imposing the prohibition (e.g., legislators) could autonomously decide that they would rather engage in the proposed exchange of refraining from imposing penalties in return for plasma centers refraining from offering compensation for plasma. Similarly, given the situation that they are in, the persons upon whom the penalties would fall (e.g., those operating plasma centers, or prospective donors) could autonomously decide that they would prefer to refrain from offering (or receiving) compensation for plasma in exchange for not having the relevant penalties imposed upon them. Moreover, the persons responsible for prohibiting compensation could also autonomously decide that they would prefer that this type of transaction (i.e., where they refrain from imposing penalties in exchange for the procurement agencies refraining from offering financial compensation) be one that is allowed rather than precluded. They could thus meet condition 2. However, if *absent such prohibition* persons operating plasma centers would autonomously decide to offer financial compensation to prospective donors then this exchange would not satisfy condition (2) for them. This is because in that case they would have autonomously decided that they would *prefer* to offer compensation rather than be prohibited from so doing. Similarly, if prospective donors would autonomously decide that they would prefer to be in a situation where they could receive compensation for their donations rather than not they, too, will fail to meet condition 2 with respect to the legislator's proposal to refrain from prosecuting them if they refrained from accepting compensation for their plasma.[42] Thus, in a situation where the offer of financial compensation for plasma is prohibited and where the plasma centers would otherwise offer such compensation and at least some donors would willingly accept it, the legislator's proposal of refraining from imposing penalties on plasma center in exchange for their refraining from offering compensation is morally impermissible. Since these empirical conditions are met the legislator's proposal is morally akin to the highwayman's proposal to refrain from shooting her victim if he surrenders his money to her.[43]

Conclusion

Persons concerned with both the moral quality of donor consent and donor well-being should thus support allowing plasma centers to offer compensation to prospective donors and oppose their being legally prohibited from doing so. This conclusion is striking – not least because it has been derived from the best argument in support of the view that offering prospective plasma donors compensation adversely affects their autonomy with respect to their acts of donation in a manner that is functionally equivalent to coercion. But it is important not to overstate what the earlier argument has established.

First, while meeting both conditions (1) and (2) required for Two-Tier Consent is necessary for a proposal and consequent exchange to be morally permissible, it does not suffice for this. The exchange might violate moral duties that are owed to third parties. The parties to an assassin contract, for example, might both meet both conditions (1) and (2). But this would not suffice to render this exchange permissible as it would violate the moral claim of the prospective victim not to be killed.[44] Second, the earlier account of the conditions that must be met for an exchange to be morally permissible are just that – conditions that must be met for a *particular* exchange to be morally permissible. The earlier argument thus does not directly support any *a priori* claim concerning the moral permissibility or otherwise of any general policy concerning donor compensation. But is (as seems plausible) the majority of commercial plasma centers and prospective donors would respectively prefer both to offer and then exchange compensation for plasma, and to receive such offers and then donate for compensation, and both would also prefer that these exchanges be allowed, then the offer of compensation for plasma donation and the consummation of exchanges motivated by this activation offer would be permissible. Conversely, if commercial plasma centers and prospective donors would prefer that offers of compensation not be prohibited then even if they abided by this prohibition and refrained from such exchange (and so satisfied condition (1) with respect to this prohibitive proposal), they would not satisfy condition (2). Their consent to refrain from (respectively) offering or receiving compensation would thus be defective and so the consummation of this prohibitive proposal (i.e., the effective prohibition of compensated plasma donation) would be morally impermissible. In practice as in theory, then, persons concerned with both the moral quality of donor consent and donor well-being should thus support allowing plasma centers to offer compensation to prospective donors and oppose their being legally prohibited from so doing.

Notes

1. See, for example, Steven Weimer, "'I Can't Eat if I Don't Plass': Impoverished Plasma Donors, Alternatives, and Autonomy," *HEC Forum* 27 (2015), 261–285. That a person's poverty could coerce her into selling her blood was assumed by Vincanne Adams, Kathleen Erwin, and Phuoc V. Le, "Public Health Works: Blood Donation in Urban China," *Social Science & Medicine* 68 (2009), 415. This view is recognized but not endorsed by Lucie White, "Does Remuneration for Plasma Compromise Autonomy?" *HEC Forum* 27 (2015), 390–391, and by Farrugia and Del Bò, "Some reflections on the Code of Ethics of the International Society of Blood Transfusion," 553.
2. The term "proposal" encompasses both threats and offers.
3. R.W. Beal and W.G. van Aken, "Gift or Good? A Contemporary Examination of the Voluntary and Commercial Aspects of Blood Donation," *Vox Sanguinis* 63, 1 (1992), 3.
4. Gilles Folléa, Erhard Seifried, and Jeroen de Wit, "Renewed Considerations on Ethical Values for Blood and Plasma Donations and Donors," *Blood Transfusion* 12, Suppl. 1 (2014), s.387. This argument has also been recognized (but not endorsed) by Alena M. Buyx, "Blood Donation, Payment, and Non-Cash Incentives: Classical Questions Drawing Renewed Interest," *Transfusion medicine and hemotherapy: offizielles Organ der Deutschen Gesellschaft fur Transfusionsmedizin und Immunhamatologie* 36, 5 (2009), 330–331.
5. To their credit Health Canada expressly notes that "'voluntary/volunteer' and 'paid' are imperfect terms to differentiate donors and the donation event, but they are used in this report to distinguish between unpaid/uncompensated/non-remunerated and paid/compensated/remunerated donors/donations. There is no suggestion that any donations are 'involuntary' in the sense of being mandatory or forced." Health Canada. *Protecting Access to Immune Globulins for Canadians*, 8.
6. See, for example, WHO, *Towards 100% Voluntary Blood Donation: A Global Framework for Action* (WHO: Geneva, 2010).
7. The terms "voluntary" and "nonvoluntary" are standard in this debate and should be considered terms of art within it. To situate them within mainstream philosophical terminology, the claim that a person is voluntary with respect to her act of donating plasma can be glossed as the claim that she is autonomous with respect to it, while the claim that a person's donation is nonvoluntary can be glossed as the claim that her autonomy with respect to her act of donation has been compromised.
8. For a discussion of coercive offers, see David Zimmerman, "Coercive Wage Offers," *Philosophy & Public Affairs* 10, 2 (1981), 121–145.
9. I will grant this claim for the sake of argument.
10. This premise is influenced by Gerald Dworkin's work on coercion. See "Acting Freely," *Nous* 4, 4 (1970), 377–378.
11. Joshua Penrod and Albert Farrugia note that lottery tickets and paid days off work are not considered to be "compensation" or incentives to donate plasma. As they rightly (and acerbically) note "[t]his is reasoning controlled

by regulatory definitional fiat." Penrod and Farrugia, "Errors and Omissions," 321. See also the discussion in Chapter 1.

12. An argument of this form has been suggested by Nicola Lacetera, "Incentives and Ethics in the Economics of Body Parts," National Bureau of Economic Research Working Paper 22673, 5. Available at: www.nber.org/papers/w22673

13. See, for example, Robert Noggle, "Autonomy and the Paradox of Self-Creation: Infinite Regresses, Finite Selves, and the Limits of Authenticity," in James Stacey Taylor, ed., *Personal Autonomy: New Essays on Personal Autonomy and Its Role in Contemporary Moral Philosophy* (Cambridge: Cambridge University Press, 2005), 88; Laura Waddell Ekstrom, "Autonomy and Personal Integration," in James Stacey Taylor, ed. *Personal Autonomy: New Essays on Personal Autonomy and Its Role in Contemporary Moral Philosophy* (Cambridge: Cambridge University Press, 2005), 145; Tom L. Beauchamp, "Who Deserves Autonomy, and Whose Autonomy Deserves Respect," in James Stacey Taylor, ed., *Personal Autonomy: New Essays on Personal Autonomy and Its Role in Contemporary Moral Philosophy* (Cambridge: Cambridge University Press, 2005), 313.

14. Harry Frankfurt's analysis of identification is often taken to be a hierarchical account of autonomy of this sort. See, for example, his "Freedom of the Will and the Concept of a Person," *The Journal of Philosophy* 68, 1 (1971), 5–20. See also Dworkin, "Acting Freely," 367–383.

15. See Irving Thalberg, "Hierarchical Analyses of Unfree Action," *Canadian Journal of Philosophy* 8, 2 (1978), 213–215.

16. A version of this argument was originally developed in James Stacey Taylor, "Autonomy, Duress, and Coercion," *Social Philosophy & Policy* 20, 2 (2003), 127–155.

17. This is a modified version of the Threshold Condition that was first developed in James Stacey Taylor, *Practical Autonomy and Bioethics* (New York: Routledge, 2009), 7.

18. This account of the Degree Condition is modified from Taylor, *Practical Autonomy and Bioethics*, 8. Note that for a person to be genuinely satisfied with a particular decision-making procedure her satisfaction must meet the same type of Threshold condition that her decision-making must meet, and so it should not be the result of the manipulation of her beliefs without her knowledge. (This entails that whether or not a person is autonomous with respect to a particular decision will not be first-person accessible, just as persons who are straightforwardly manipulated could suffer from diminutions in their autonomy without knowing this.) Second, the account of autonomy that is developed here is a *political* account: The essential question is whether the person whose autonomy is in question is the font of the decision (desire, action), or whether this is someone else. Thus, if a person has been subject to manipulation at either the decision-making level or the satisfaction level then (given the failure of the Threshold Condition, insofar as this applies to both of these levels) she will suffer from a diminution in her autonomy with respect to her decisions provided that this manipulation results in someone else being the font of the putative satisfaction of the conditions for her to be autonomous with respect to them. (Hence, the motivation for holding that the Threshold condition must be met at the level of satisfaction is the same as that which motivated it at the level of decisions.) I thank Steve Weimer for helpful discussion on these points. He was right that my initial versions of these conditions were too loose!

19. This is a modified version of the Tracking Condition that I first developed in Taylor, *Practical Autonomy and Bioethics*, 11.

20. This is not quite right, although it suffices for the purposes of the analysis here. A person who is coerced into performing an action will not (typically) abdicate all control over her actions to her coercer. Instead, she will still (tacitly) retain the option of refusing to obey his commands if she believes that it would be better for her to resist his attempt to coerce her rather than perform the actions that he requires. Thus, rather than ceding all control over her actions to her coerced she will cede all control over her actions provided that they are from a particular set of actions that she would be willing to perform to avoid the threatened penalty.

21. I do not mean to imply that every proponent of the Argument from Coercion will advance this Argument from Force, only that some might.

22. This argument is expressly rejected by Health Canada. See Health Canada, *Protecting Access to Immune Globulins for Canadians*, 8.

23. This is a version of the "double bind" discussed by Margaret Jane Radin. Radin was concerned with the effects that allowing the sales of certain goods would have upon the personhood of those who sold them but recognized that attempts to protect their personhood by precluding such sales "might deprive a class of poor and oppressed people of the opportunity to have more money with which to buy adequate food, shelter, and healthcare in the market, and hence deprive them of a better chance to lead a humane life." Margaret Jane Radin, *Contested Commodities* (Cambridge, MA: Harvard University Press, 1996), 125.

24. See, for example, Robert Young, "The Value of Autonomy," *The Philosophical Quarterly* 32, 126 (1982), 35–44.

25. An earlier version of this argument was developed in Taylor, *Practical Autonomy and Bioethics*, 144–145.

26. Instead, its value is derivative from the value of the outcome that was a result of its exercise.

27. This is not surprising, for if it was true that persons should never compromise their autonomy for any perceived increase in their well-being persons should never, for example, agree to be directed by others in exchange for compensation. This would undermine the moral legitimacy of most employment contracts. And this is absurd.

28. On the latter issue see, for example, James Stacey Taylor, *Death, Posthumous Harm, and Bioethics* (New York: Routledge, 2012), 42–47.

29. Here I agree with Warnock, when she writes that "No one would suggest that selling your kidney [or plasma] is something you do like gasping or shuddering or letting out a cry." ("Will liberty lead us to an internal market?", 3).

30. This example is adapted from Joseph Raz's example of "The Man in the Pit" – although Raz uses his version of this example to argue (erroneously) that autonomy requires an "adequate" range of options. *The Morality of Freedom* (Oxford: Clarendon Press, 1986), 373–374.

31. Although I have used the plural here as far as I know the only proponent of this argument – which is the best argument available to those who oppose donor compensation out of a moral concern with donor autonomy – is myself. I can thus say with confidence that I do not make the mistake I identify earlier.

32. Subject to the caveat noted earlier, in note 20.

33. This argument does not show that providing compensation is morally objectionable, only that offering to provide it could be. If a person would have

been willing to donate whether or not compensation was offered, then she would have initiated the donation. It would thus be her, and not the plasma center, that was directing her act of donation for she would not have ceded any control over her actions to it. She would be in the same position as a person who performed the actions that her coercer required of her, not because she wished to avoid the threatened penalty but because she had independently of his threat decided to perform them.

34. See Daniel Lyons, "Welcome Threats and Coercive Offers," *Philosophy* 50, 194 (1975), 436.
35. My focus here is on the moral permissibility of the consummation of a proposal. I am leaving to one side the question of whether certain offers could be wrong in themselves (e.g., professional advancement for sexual favors) even if they are not accepted.
36. An early version of this argument was developed in James Stacey Taylor, "How Not to Argue for Markets, or, Why the Argument from Mutually Beneficial Exchange Fails," *Journal of Social Philosophy* 48, 2 (2017), 165–179.
37. See, for example, Ian Maitland, "The Great Non-Debate Over International Sweatshops," *British Academy of Management Annual Conference Proceedings* (September 1997), 240–265; Matt Zwolinski, "The Ethics of Price Gouging," *Business Ethics Quarterly* 18, 3 (2008), 351; Gerald Dworkin, "Markets and Morals: The Case for Organ Sales," in Gerald Dworkin, ed., *Morality, Harm, and the Law* (Boulder, CO: Westview Press, 1994), 156, and Richard A. Posner, "The Ethics and Economics of Enforcing Contracts of Surrogate Motherhood," *Journal of Contemporary Health Law and Policy* 5 (1989), 22–23.
38. A proponent of this approach to defending markets in certain goods and services cannot appeal to the claim that those proposed exchanges that are morally permissible (e.g., those that involve lucrative job offers) can be distinguished from those that are morally impermissible (e.g., "Your money or your life!") on the grounds that the former transactions will be entered into voluntarily by both parties while the latter will not be. As argued earlier both of these transactions could be functionally equivalent with respect to the autonomy, the voluntariness, of the person to whom the exchange was proposed. She could also not simply hold that those exchanges that a person was coerced into performing would be impermissible and those that she entered into freely would be permissible, for this would be *ad hoc* – an account must be given as to *why* coerced exchanges are impermissible.
39. James Tobin, "On Limiting the Domain of Inequality," *Journal of Law and Economics* 13, 2 (1970), 269; Christopher Freiman, "Vote Markets," *Australasian Journal of Philosophy* 92, 4 (2014), 761.
40. There is a complication here: that under these conditions no voter would have a reason to cast her vote. But if this were so some voters would be motivated to cast their votes as they could believe that they would now be pivotal. This, in turn, would lead back to the view that there would be no reason to cast votes as none would be pivotal. It is thus indeterminate as to whether or not a rational self-interested person would vote. However, this complication can be put to one side for since this indeterminacy would be equally spread among the voting public it is likely that given the greater number of Poor voters the Poor Party could always be expected to win.
41. See Taylor, "How Not to Argue for Markets," 165–179.
42. Evidence for the existence of donors with this preference ranking is given in Chapter 5.

43. In fact, the legislator's offer here would be *worse* on consequentialist grounds as it imposes unnecessary costs on third parties in a way that the highwayman's offer would not. The prohibition of compensation for plasma would either lead to some patients not receiving the medical products that they need and would otherwise secure, or to these being costlier. Persons who prohibit financial compensation for plasma are in this respect morally worse than street thugs.

44. It is also possible that a failure to meet condition 2 would not preclude an exchange from being morally permissible – in which case meeting both conditions would fail to be necessary for an exchange to be morally permissible. Consider a case in which A and B were about to participate in an exchange in which both conditions were met. C then makes a prohibitive proposal to B to preclude the exchange from taking place on the grounds that B's participation in this exchange would preclude her from meeting her moral obligation to D (e.g., she is using the money that she must repay D to buy a new jacket). If C's interference with B's actions is legitimate, then her prohibitive offer (and the resulting transaction between her and B) would be one in which the failure of B to meet both conditions does not preclude the exchange in which she participates with B from being morally legitimate. Given this, condition 2 should be modified so that a person's endorsement or rejection of the type of exchange was based on (i) her concern for her own well-being and (ii) where this concern did not take illegitimate precedence over any prior moral obligations that she might have. With this modification in place, B would not fail to meet condition 2 and so C's prohibitive offer would not be impermissible on this account of consent (although it might be impermissible for other reasons).

4   Exploitation

Introduction

It is widely held that compensating donors for their plasma will exploit them.[1] Carlo Petrini, for example, worries that compensated donors "could too easily be exploited,"[2] while Adrian Walsh recognizes the force of the worry that compensated plasma donors who sell "in desperate circumstances" could be exploited.[3] Slonim, Wang, and Garbarino hold that "the potential exploitation of donors" is "the major ethical consideration" that arises when the question of paying donors for blood is raised – a point that can be readily generalized to the question of whether donors should be compensated for donating plasma.[4] These academic concerns with the possible exploitation of plasma donors are echoed by the WHO which states that to avoid the exploitation of donors they should not be compensated.[5] Worries about the exploitation of plasma donors are not only widespread but are also long-standing – and have had considerable influence in shaping both the theory and practice of plasma collection. As Anne-Maree Farrell notes, in the 1970s, "evidence of the exploitative plasma collection practices engaged in by the for-profit practices . . . served to intensify the importance of . . . professional belief in VNRBD [Voluntary Non-Remunerated Blood Donation]."[6]

Yet despite the long-standing and widespread concern that compensating plasma donors would exploit them, the expression of this concern is rarely accompanied by supporting argument. And when discussions of donor exploitation actually do move beyond mere expressions of concern to offer arguments they rarely engage with the relevant philosophical literature. As a result of this, they are often based on an underinformed view of what exploitation is. For example, in arguing that plasma donors would not be exploited "in well-regulated environments" M.W. Skinner et al. write that "donors could potentially be exploited by failing to adequately screen and monitor their health or by giving them insufficient information upon which to make an informed decision about donation."[7] But although a failure to "adequately screen and monitor" donors' health or a failure to secure their informed consent to donate

DOI: 10.4324/9781003263913-5

might be wrongful neither are in themselves exploitative. Neither necessarily involves the unfair treatment of donors – and it is the view that a transaction is unfair that lies at the heart of the claim that it is exploitative.[8] Similarly, Vida Panitch and Lendell Chad Horne assert that it is sufficient for a transaction to be exploitative that the exploiter "mislead or coerce the other party, thus undermining the extent to which the other party can meaningfully be said to give consent to the arrangement."[9] But while misleading or coercing one's trading partner into agreeing to transact with one is (*prima facie*) wrongful, such acts would not in themselves be exploitative – again, because neither would necessarily lead to an unfair transaction.[10]

In this chapter and the next, I will take up arms against this sea of troubles with the aim of ending them. To do so I will develop and defend an account of exploitation that both captures standard intuitions as to when a transaction is exploitative and also explains why these transactions are wrongful. With this in hand, I will be in a position to determine whether current practices of donor compensation are exploitative. I will argue in the next chapter that neither the commercial plasma centers in the United States nor those that operate in those European countries that allow compensated donation currently exploit their donors. (Note that since centers in Europe are required by law to follow compensation models that differ from those in the United States the answer to the question of whether these two sets of centers exploit their donors will be independent of each other.) Given that the (largely undefended) orthodoxy is that the practice of compensating donors is exploitative, this conclusion alone is worth the price of admission to these two chapters.

But I do not stop there. I also argue that prohibiting donor compensation leads the *non-compensating* plasma centers that operate in situations where compensation is prohibited to exploit some of their donors. In particular, such non-compensating plasma centers exploit two subsets of their donors. They exploit those who would donate plasma whether or not they received compensation for this but who would prefer to receive compensation. And they exploit those who would prefer not to donate plasma but who would do so if they believed that donations were necessary to avoid a shortage relative to medical need. Thus, a genuine concern with avoiding the exploitation of plasma donors should lead one to oppose prohibiting donor compensation.

An Analysis of Exploitation

As with the arguments discussed in the previous chapter, the argument from exploitation begins with the observation that plasma donors are often economically impoverished.[11] It then continues with the observation that while plasma donors are paid relatively little for their donations, plasma companies enjoy significant profits.[12] These observations are taken to justify the claim that the donors are exploited. With this claim in hand, it is concluded that compensated donation should be prohibited to protect prospective donors from exploitation.[13]

But while this argument is widely deployed a few moments' thought reveals that it is very strange indeed. If the concern is that plasma centers that compensate their donors exploit them by securing their plasma at a low cost relative to the profits that they will make from it the conclusion should not be that they should be required to lower the level of compensation that they offer to zero (i.e., compensation is prohibited). Instead, the conclusion should be that the compensation offered to donors should be *higher* so that they receive a more equitable share of the profits that are derived from their plasma.[14] As Alan Wertheimer has noted, the oddity of this conclusion indicates that a concern with something other than exploitation might be the driving force behind arguments of this type: That while exploitation is the expressed concern the real concern is that the donors are receiving monetary compensation for something that should not be monetarily alienable.[15] This view – that the social meaning of certain goods and services morally precludes them from being exchanged for money – will be addressed in Chapters 6 and 7. But it is also possible that some who conclude that payment for certain goods and services is morally wrong are genuinely concerned with exploitation. If they consider exploitation to be a great moral wrong and they believe that there is little to no chance of donors receiving what they would consider to be fair compensation for their donations they might support the prohibition of compensation on the grounds that this is the only practical way to protect donors from exploitation.

To address this concern, I must first identify when C exploits X. At first sight, the answer to this seems obvious: C will exploit X whenever the price that C charges X for the good or service that he sells to her is unjustly high. (Or, conversely, that the price that C pays X for the good or service that he acquires from her is unjustly low.) This answer is both unhelpful and helpful. It is unhelpful because it simply changes the question of when C exploits X to the question of when the price that C charges X is unjustly high. But it is helpful in that this change makes it clear that the question of whether C exploits X is distinct from the question of what a just price for C's goods or services should be. Establishing that C exploits X – that he charges her a price that is unjustly high – can be done without establishing what the just price is. We only need to establish that the price that C charged X was higher than that which was just.

To determine when the price that C charges X was unjustly high – and hence that he exploited her – let us consider a series of examples.[16]

> Situation 1: A, B, and C wish to exchange with X. A, B, C are corn growers; X is buying corn to eat. A tornado wipes out the crops of A and B but not of C. C now charges a much higher price to X than

she would have charged before A and B were removed from the market. Some would claim that C exploited X; that the higher price that she charged for her corn was unjust.

Situation 2: As before, A, B, and C wish to sell corn to X who is buying it to eat. C coerces A and B out of the market by threatening them with harm if they continue to compete with her. Upon their exit from the market, she can now charge a much higher price to X.

If C exploited X in Situation 1 then she would also have exploited X in Situation 2. Just as the manner of the destruction of the crops of A and B in Situation 1 is immaterial (all that matters is this enabled C to charge X a much higher price) so too is it immaterial that they were removed from the market by the successful threats of C.

But it is not clear that C exploited X in Situation 1. Consider

Situation 3: Pests destroy some (but not all) of the corn grown by A and B; C's corn is unaffected. The price of corn rises as a result. This greatly benefits C who has the same amount of corn to sell but who can now charge a much higher price for it – indeed, she can now charge the same price as she charged X in Situation 1. However, it adversely affects X who buys corn to eat from C at the higher price. (A and B are financially unaffected; they have less corn to sell but the price increase makes up for this.)

In this situation, C does not exploit X. When he buys from her, she simply charges him the same rate that A or B would have charged him. It is merely unfortunate for X that this rate is higher than it was before the crops of A and B were afflicted by pests. Since the price that C charged X in Situation 3 is the same as she charged in Situation 1, the question of whether she exploited him cannot be decided by appeal to price alone. (Recall, while there is some question as to whether she exploited him in Situation 1 she did not do so in Situation 3, even though the price she charges in both situations is the same.) It might be tempting to hold that C did not exploit X in Situation 3 because he had a choice of from whom to buy corn. But this cannot explain why X was not exploited by C in Situation 3. If there was a perfectly competitive market for corn in Situation 3, A, B, and C would all charge the same price for corn. While X could then choose from whom he bought the corn, this would be a choice with no meaning.[17] Moreover, consider

Situation 4: C operates a towing company in a mountainous area with little population and no cell phone reception. In the winter, she spends her time driving along the main roads looking for people whose vehicles have broken down so that she can offer to tow them to the nearest town. She charges a very high price for this rescue service. When stranded motorists complain that her prices are exploitative she responds by telling them that she finds very few people in need of her services for only a few people break down. She also points out that were she not to be looking for stranded motorists she would be earning money by towing people in town, or by plowing snow. To offset her opportunity costs she charges the few people that she finds high prices for her services. Sometimes the motorists tell her that they will take their chances that another towing company will come by. C informs them that she has no competition. The other towing companies in town have decided not to compete with her because the higher the number of towing companies that are out looking for stranded motorists, the lower the chance that any one company will find enough stranded motorists to make a profit. When the skeptical motorists protest that they would pay almost anything to be towed out C responds that that might be true. But she does not charge "almost anything" because if prices rose to that level, then it would be worthwhile for other companies to compete with her even given the low number of motorists that get stranded. Thus, while her prices seem high, they only cover her costs together with a (slightly) higher profit than she could make by working in town.

In Situation 4, the stranded motorists have no choice from whom to buy towing services. But C's argument that she does not exploit them is persuasive. (Note that this argument does not claim that she does not exploit them because they are – at least *ex ante* – made better off by transacting with her than not. In Situation 2, X is made better off by transacting with C than he would be were he not to do this and yet he is still exploited by her. An exploitative transaction could still be mutually advantageous.) An exploitative transaction thus cannot be identified by appeal to the price alone (i.e., it is "clearly too high," and hence exploitative). Nor can it be identified by the lack of choices that one of the parties to the transaction has. (The mere fact that a vendor has a *de facto* monopoly over a particular good or service does not thereby render her sales of it exploitative.) But now consider a variant on Situation 4:

> Situation 5: C operates her emergency towing service as before. But this time she charges far more than she did in Situation 4. When a stranded economist noted that it would not be long before her high profits would attract competition, she responded that this is why she has a clause in her towing contract that to receive her services the motorist must agree to say only that he paid her what he would have paid in Situation 4 – an amount that is much lower than the actual price. C widely publicizes the lower (false) charge and so dissuades competition.

Just as C exploits X in Situation 2 so too does she exploit the stranded motorists in Situation 5. In both cases, she acts to eliminate the actual or prospective competition that she would face in the marketplace so that the supply of the goods or services that she provides is artificially low enabling her to charge higher prices. But it is not necessary for C to eliminate her competition to engage in exploitation. Consider

> Situation 6: C is drinking in a bar when a well-known local criminal enters. The criminal places a dollar on the bar and tells the barman that he is buying drinks for everyone in the house – and that he wants change. The barman recognizes the implicit threat and serves people what they order. C orders an expensive whisky – making it clear that she wants "a triple."

C here takes advantage of the criminal's act to exploit the barman: She acts so that he will provide a good to her at a lower price than he would have otherwise been able to charge.[18] While Situation 6 differs from Situations 2 and 5 in that C does not act to eliminate her competition it does share an important feature with them: An agent acted to bring it about that the price of the good or service that was the subject of the transaction did not reflect the actual relationship between its supply and the demand for it. It is tempting to conclude from this that C exploits X to the degree that C secures a benefit from a transaction with X as the result of an agent (either C or someone else) acting to bring it about that the price of the good or service that is the subject of the transaction does not reflect the actual relationship between its supply and the demand for it. But this will not do. C could reduce the price at which he is willing to sell a good to X below that which would reflect the relationship between its supply and the demand for it, knowing that X could not afford the good at the higher (market) price and that he (C) would still make a small profit on the sale. In this case, C would not have exploited X but would have acted magnanimously toward her. To capture the core idea that an exploiter will benefit at the expense of the exploited, a further element must be introduced into the earlier account: C exploits X to the degree that the benefit that C secures from a transaction with X is the result of an agent (either C or someone else) acting so that the price of the good or service that is the subject of the transaction does not reflect the actual relationship between its supply and the demand for it *and* where the benefit C secures is greater than that which she would have received had this interference in the price signal concerning the good or service in question not occurred with C securing this additional benefit at the expense of X.

Before moving to defend this market-based account of exploitation, four observations are in order. First, on this account of exploitation C does not exploit X in Situation 1. This might render this account of exploitation implausible for some. I will thus address this issue more fully in the following when this account of exploitation is defended. Second, this account of exploitation is limited to situations where the person who is exploited is able to consent to the transaction in which he is exploited in the sense required for him to normatively authorize it.[19] It does not cover cases where a person is said to have been exploited as a result of his exploiter taking advantage of his cognitive deficiencies (e.g., a child who has been "exploited" by an adult who takes advantage of his failure to understand the terms of the contract that he signed). Third, this account of exploitation entails that the imposition of price ceilings and price floors could lead to (possibly blameless) exploitation. This would occur if they rendered the price of the good or service affected by them unresponsive to the actual relationship that holds between its supply and the demand for it with the resulting unresponsive price providing a greater benefit to one party to the transaction than she would have received had these price controls not been in place. Finally, it is possible for someone to exploit another blamelessly. This might occur if the exploiter was unaware that he was engaging in exploitation. Consider again the situation where a criminal places a dollar on a bar and informs the barman that he is using this to buy drinks for everyone in the bar. After he does this, a stranger to the neighborhood enters the bar and orders a drink. (Call this variation on Situation 6 "The Stranger in the Bar.") If, at the behest of the criminal, the barman serves him free of charge then he would have met the conditions outlined earlier for him to have exploited the barman. But because he was unaware of the situation, he would not be blameworthy for accepting the drink. He would have blamelessly exploited the barman. Blameless exploitation might also occur if the exploitation is morally justified. If the imposition of minimum wage levels is morally justified all-things-considered to ensure that at least some of the working poor can secure what is held to be a reasonable standard of living, then the workers who received this minimum wage (and who would not have done so absent their being required) would blamelessly exploit their employers.

Defending This Account of Exploitation

The claim that C does not exploit X in Situation 1 might be found by some to so implausible as to provide a reason to reject this account of exploitation. In response, it should be noted that the claim that C does not exploit X in this situation does not imply that she does not wrong him in some other way. If C had a moral obligation to X to provide him with corn, then she would wrong him if she charged him for it.[20] But the wrong that she would do to him would be that of the misappropriation of his goods (i.e., the corn to which he had a moral right) through ransom, not exploitation. If this was the case, then it would be C's act of charging X for a good that was already his by right that would be wrongful – not her act of charging a price that was higher than it would have been had A and B been able to compete with her in the marketplace.

One might, however, insist that C exploited X in Situation 1. To support this claim, one would have to provide an analysis of why the price that C charged X would be exploitative. To say that this price would be "unfair" would clearly be unhelpful on its own for then an account of what constituted an "unfair" exchange would have to be provided. And none of the obvious accounts of what would constitute an unfair exchange is plausible. The view that an exchange will only be fair if both parties to it receive the same amount of benefit from it would render almost every mutually advantageous voluntary exchange "unfair." Moreover, given the low profit margins enjoyed by most retailers, this view would have the counterintuitive result that consumers are routinely unfair to the corporations with whom they transact. Imagine, for example, that the grocery store Kroger has an operating profit margin of c. 1.5% on its typical product.[21] It is likely that Kroger's customers value the items that they buy from it at more than 1.5% above the price that they pay. If so, then on this view of what counts as a "fair" transaction, Kroger is routinely exploited by its customers. But this is implausible. A less restrictive alternative to this view is that a "fair" transaction is one in which each party receives a "comparable" benefit from it. But what this view gains in plausibility when compared to the view that the parties should receive equal benefits it loses in vagueness. It is not clear what would constitute a (nonarbitrary) "comparable" benefit. This view also has counterintuitive results. If the stranded motorist in Situation 5 were a diabetic who had run out of insulin and needed to get to the nearest town to replenish his supply, he might receive an incomparably greater value from his transaction with C than she did even given the (uncompetitively) high price that she charged him to tow him there. But it would be odd to say that in this case the diabetic motorist exploited C. Recognizing the difficulties that beset any *a priori* specification of fairness, one might be tempted to offer an *a posteriori* account: A fair transaction would be that which was conducted at the usual market price, free from force and fraud. (Or, less restrictively, a fair transaction is that which is conducted within certain parameters that are indexed to the usual market rate.) But in taking the normal market price for a good or service to be normative, this approach illicitly moves from a descriptive claim ("the normal market price for G is P") to a normative claim ("the fair price for G is P," or "the fair price for G is P, plus or minus some amount Q"). It is also unclear how the "normal market price" should be determined. The most plausible candidate for this would be that which held just prior to the transaction whose fairness is in question.[22] But this price is – like the allegedly unfair price that follows it – simply the result of the relationship between the supply of the good in question and the demand for it. It is thus unclear why this has any normative significance: Why this should be considered the "normal" ("fair") price and that which follows it an "abnormal" ("unfair") price? It is also unclear how a principled account of which price prior to the allegedly exploitative transaction could be provided. Consider again Situation 3. In the year prior to Situation 3 (i.e., before pests afflicted the crops of A and B), the price of corn would have been lower than it was in Situation 3. If we take this as the baseline, then the price that C changed X in this situation would have been unfair; she would have exploited him. But if the pests continue to afflict the crops of A and B over the course of several years and so the price of corn remains high it is not clear why the new higher price should not be taken to be the normal market price. If it is, then it is not clear why the initial higher price (in Situation 3) was unfair simply because it occurred after a lower price was being charged. If, however, the lower price continues to be taken to be the normal market price then this approach starts to appear *ad hoc*, with the lower price being normative for no other reason than it is lower. A defender of the view that the "normal" market price is normative might respond by noting that in the first year(s) of the higher price X would be worse off paying them than he would in subsequent years as he would not have time to plan to accommodate what was then an unexpected cost and so he would be worse off in those years with the same price than he would be in subsequent years. Hence, she might continue, the lower price should initially be normative, with the higher price becoming normative as the years pass. But even if this claim concerning the differential effects on X were true this does not show that C exploited X (or wronged him in any other way) by charging him the higher price in the initial year(s). It merely shows that X was worse off in those years. The mere fact that X was worse off as a result of a combination of his circumstances and C's actions does now show that C thereby wronged him (by exploiting him).

Conclusion

The aforementioned defense of this market-based account of exploitation has been indirect, showing that the rejection of it on the grounds that C did exploit X in Situation 1 will itself be faced with serious theoretical difficulties. But showing that the view that C exploited X in Situation 1 faces theoretical difficulties (i.e., showing that the objection to this account of exploitation is itself problematic) does not show that the earlier analysis of exploitation should be accepted. To support this account, then, some of its positive qualities should be outlined. First (apart from the contentious Situation 1) this analysis gives the intuitively right answers in each of the other situations that it considers. Second, in holding that C exploits X when C receives additional benefits from X as a result of agential interference with the price of the good or service that is the subject of the transaction, this analysis captures the worry (identified by Wertheimer as the focus of the concern about exploitation) that resources from X have been transferred to C through force.[23] Finally, by retaining the focus on the justice of prices reached through market means, this analysis is firmly within the mainstream tradition of analyses of exploitation. This should be emphasized before moving to apply this analysis to the question of whether plasma donors are exploited by the plasma centers that offer them compensation. This is because the conclusion that will be drawn from this application of this analysis will be the opposite of that which is now drawn in discussions of compensated donation: That not only are donors not exploited by the plasma centers that compensate them but that the prohibition of compensation will lead to the exploitation of some *uncompensated* donors. I will turn to these issues in the next chapter.

Notes

1. See, for example, Pablo Rodriguez del Pozo, "Paying Donors and the Ethics of Blood Supply," *Journal of Medical Ethics* 20 (1994), 33; P. Flanagan, "Self-Sufficiency in Plasma Supply – Achievable and Desirable?" *ISBT Science Series* 12 (2017), 484; Jerry F. Brown et al., "Apheresis for Collection of Ebola Convalescent Plasma in Liberia," *Journal of Clinical Apheresis* 32, 3 (2017), 180; Beal and Aken, "Gift or Good?" 3; Keown, "The Gift of Blood in Europe," 98–99.
2. Carlo Petrini, "Production of Plasma-Derived Medicinal Products: Ethical Implications for Blood Donations and Donors," *Blood Transfusion* 12, Supp. 1 (2014); s390.
3. Adrian Walsh, "Compensation for Blood Plasma Donation as a *Distinctive* Ethical Hazard: Reformulating the Commodification Objection," *HEC Forum* 27, 4 (2015), 413.
4. Robert Slonim, Carmen Wang, and Ellen Garbarino, "The Market for Blood," *Journal of Economic Perspectives* 28, 2 (2014), 185.
5. WHO, "The Rome Declaration on Achieving Self-Sufficiency in Safe Blood and Blood Products, based on Voluntary Non-Remunerated Donation," www.avis.it/userfiles/file/RomeDeclarationSelf-SufficiencySafeBloodBlood ProductsVNRD.pdf. See also WHO Expert Group, "Expert Consensus Statement on Achieving Self-Sufficiency in Safe Blood and Blood Products Based on Voluntary Non-Remunerated Blood Donation (VNRBD)," *Vox Sanguinis* 103, 4 (2012), 339. This Consensus Statement explicitly refers to blood donors but since they mention plasma donors immediately before this claim it is clear that they intend it to apply to them also. (The WHO Expert Group states that donors should not be compensated to avoid exploitation in a section of their "Consensus Statement" which begins with the observation that the "Oviedo Convention on Human Rights and Biomedicine of 1997 explicitly prohibits any financial gain from the human body and its parts.") Immediately after this they state that "[p]revention of the commercialization of donation of blood, plasma and cellular components and exploitation of blood donors are important ethical principles on which a national blood system should be based," thereby giving the impression that these ethical concerns were raised by the Oviedo Convention (WHO Expert Group, "Expert Consensus Statement," 339). But the Oviedo Convention provides no reason

to support its assertion that "[t]he human body and its parts shall not, as such, give rise to financial gain." Oviedo Convention, "Chapter 7, Article 21," Available at: www.coe.int/en/web/conventions/full-list/-/conventions/rms/090000168007cf98.

6. Farrell, *The Politics of Blood*, 82. Farrell is referring here to collection practices in the 1970s, not today. Note, too, that she provides no actual examples of donor exploitation to support her assertion.

7. M. W. Skinner et al., "Risk-Based Decision Making and Ethical Considerations in Donor Compensation for Plasma-Derived Medicinal Products," *Transfusion* 56, 11 (2016), 2891.

8. Alan Wertheimer, *Exploitation* (Princeton: Princeton University Press, 1996), 247. See also Stephen Wilkinson's account of exploitation as involving a "disparity of value"; Stephen Wilkinson, *Bodies for Sale: Ethics and Exploitation in the Human Body Trade* (New York: Routledge, 2003), 34.

9. Vida Panitch and Lendell Chad Horne, "Paying for Plasma: Commodification, Exploitation, and Canada's Plasma Shortage," *Canadian Journal of Bioethics* 2, 2 (2019), 3.

10. Panitch and Horne recognize that one party to a transaction would exploit another if "they deny the other party something they are truly owed, a fair share of the benefits of the exchange," dubbing this "the *fairness* criterion." (Panitch and Horne, "Paying for Plasma," 3). But they hold this to be an independent condition of the "*consent* criterion" outlined earlier, thus mistakenly conflating the wrongs of deception (or manipulation) and coercion with that of exploitation. Problems with approaches such as the fairness criterion will be outlined in the following.

11. See, for example, H. Luke Shaffer and Analidis Ochoa, "How Blood-Plasma Companies Target the Poorest Americans," *The Atlantic* (March 15, 2018). As with the discussion in Chapter 3, the following reconstruction of the argument from exploitation is highly charitable. Those who draw on the claim that donors are exploited to justify the prohibition of donor compensation rarely offer an argument as developed as this, often simply asserting that donors are exploited.

12. Panitch and Horne, for example, express concern about "allowing a private company to profit from Canada's blood supply." Panitch and Horne, "Paying for Plasma," 1.

13. See WHO Expert Group, "Expert Consensus Statement," 339.

14. This is noted by Panitch and Horne, "Paying for Plasma," 3. It might be tempting to argue against prohibition in the following way: (1) The opponents of compensated donation claim that compensated donors are exploited as they are securing an unfairly low level of compensation relative to the profits reaped by the commercial plasma centers to whom they donate. (2) Plasma centers that accept uncompensated donations in legal regimes that prohibit compensation provide less benefits to their donors than do commercial plasma centers that compensate their donors. Hence, if the concern with exploitation is that there is an unjust distribution of burdens one should hold that agencies that do not compensate their donors are more exploitative than those who do. But the temptation to argue in this way should be resisted *unless* it can be established that the benefits that the non-compensating centers reap from the donations that they receive are as disproportionate to the benefits that their donors receive from donating as are those secured by the commercial agencies when compared with those of their donors.

15. Wertheimer, *Exploitation*, 101–102. Wertheimer makes this observation in the context of arguments from exploitation leveled against commercial surrogate pregnancy.

16. For the same of simplicity, these examples will take C to be exploiting X by charging her an unjustly high price. It is also possible that C might be exploiting X by paying her an unjustly low price.
17. Strictly, X would not be choosing, he would merely be picking.
18. The criminal coerces the barman into providing the bar's patrons drinks at lower prices than he would have been able to charge for them; the patrons that take advantage of the criminal's coercion of the barman exploit him. The criminal thus does not exploit the barman on behalf of the patrons, as Wertheimer would claim (Wertheimer, *Exploitation*, 210) but makes his exploitation by them possible.
19. See the discussion in the previous chapter.
20. Stephen Wilkinson, "The Exploitation Argument Against Commercial Surrogacy," *Bioethics* 17, 2 (2003), 178.
21. The operating profit is defined as "sales less costs and expenses, excluding net interest expenses." See Jerry Hausman and Ephraim Leibtag, "Consumer Benefits from Increased Competition in Shopping Outlets: Measuring the Effect of Wal-Mart," *Journal of Applied Econometrics* 22 (2007), 1173. That Kroger's (overall) operating profit was c. 1.5% (in 2004) is taken from ibid., Figure 2.
22. Moving further back in time leads to odd results. The "normal market price" for a home computer, for example, has dropped precipitously over the last two decades. Does this mean that consumers are now exploiting sellers, or does it mean that in the past sellers were exploiting consumers? Should this be indexed to 2000 (in which case consumers are exploiting sellers) or to 2020 (in which case sellers in 2000 were exploiting consumers)?
23. Wertheimer, *Exploitation*, 27.

5   Donor Exploitation

Introduction

In the previous chapter, I outlined and defended an account of exploitation that was intended to capture how this concept is used both in lay discussion and in philosophical debate. It is now time to draw upon this account of exploitation to assess the widespread claim that donors who accept compensation for their plasma are thereby exploited. As with the discussion of informed consent in Chapter 2, and the discussion of donor autonomy and authoritative consent in Chapter 3, this discussion of donor exploitation will lead to surprising results. It will, first, lead to the conclusion that the commercial plasma centers that currently operate in the United States and Europe that offer compensation to their donors do not thereby exploit them. But it will also lead to the striking conclusion that plasma centers that operate in situations where donor compensation is prohibited exploit some of their donors. The moral concern to avoid donor exploitation should thus lead one to encourage donor compensation and oppose its prohibition.

Exploitation and Plasma Donation

On the analysis of exploitation that I developed in the previous chapter, plasma donors will be exploited by the centers to which they donate iff (1) either the plasma center to which they donated or a third party acted so that the amount of compensation that they received did not reflect the relationship between the supply of plasma and the demand for it and (2) where the benefit that the plasma center receives from the procurement of plasma as a result of the interference noted in (1) is greater than it would have received had this interference not occurred, with this additional benefit being secured at the expense of the donors. Consider, for example, a situation in which a plasma center that offers donor compensation is granted a legal monopoly over the procurement of plasma within a particular city. This monopoly enables it to offer lower amounts of compensation than it would have needed to offer to secure donors had it had

DOI: 10.4324/9781003263913-6

to compete with other compensating plasma centers. Since its donors would have preferred to have received the higher level of compensation that they would have received had this monopoly not been in place the plasma center benefits from it at their expense. This monopoly thus enables this center to exploit its donors. Similarly, competing compensating plasma centers would exploit their donors if they colluded to fix the level of compensation that they offer at an amount lower than that which they would have to offer were they to compete with each other.

Just as it is possible that plasma centers that compensate their donors could exploit them so too is it possible that plasma centers that did *not* offer compensation could exploit their donors. Consider, for example, donors who would prefer to receive financial compensation for their donations but who would donate even if they were not offered this. If the provision of financial compensation were legally prohibited these donors would still donate plasma to a center that did not offer compensation. If the relationship between the supply of plasma and the demand for it was such that absent the prohibition of financial compensation for plasma donation the level of compensation that would be offered would be greater than zero, then the amount of compensation that this plasma center would offer ($0) for plasma would fail to accurately reflect this relationship. Moreover, the benefit that this non-compensating plasma center would gain from the plasma that was donated to it by these donors would be greater than that which it would have received had this interference in the price signal not occurred. With this interference in the price signal, it would not financially compensate its donors. Were this interference to be absent, however, it would compensate its donors. The center recognizes that its donors would prefer to receive compensation rather than not, and consequently believes that to secure plasma it would need to offer donor compensation.[1] This additional benefit (i.e., the difference between $0 and the amount of financial compensation that the centers would otherwise offer to secure their donors' plasma) is secured at the expense of the donors who would have preferred to have been compensated rather than not.[2] This plasma center would thus have exploited these donors.

There is a second class of donors that is vulnerable to exploitation by plasma centers that are prohibited from compensating their donors. These are donors who would only donate plasma if they believed that there is a shortage of supply relative to demand. Some of these donors believe that if financial compensation is not offered for plasma donations, then there will be a shortage of supply relative to demand. This subset of these donors thus donate when financial compensation for plasma is prohibited. The plasma centers that are prohibited from offering compensation to this subset of donors will benefit from securing their plasma. Since these donors will donate when compensation is prohibited the plasma centers to whom they donate their plasma secure the benefit of receiving it as a result of the prohibition of compensation. Were this prohibition not to be in place, they would not benefit from receiving these donors' plasma. The benefit that these plasma centers receive from these donors is thus greater in a situation where compensated donation is prohibited than it would be in a situation where this is allowed. The plasma centers secure this benefit at the expense of these donors. In donating these donors incur costs that they would have preferred not to have incurred. They do not wish to donate plasma *simpliciter*. They only wish to donate in a situation where they believe there will be a shortage of plasma owing to the prohibition of compensation. They prefer that there is no shortfall and they do not have to donate. If these donors *do* donate, then they will be doing something that they would prefer they did not have to do. If they donate, then, the plasma centers will benefit from their donations, they will benefit from them to a greater extent than had donor compensation not been prohibited (as they would then not occur), and they will benefit at these donors' expense. These donors will thus be exploited by the plasma centers to whom they donate their plasma.

Plasma centers that are prohibited from compensating their donors but which continue to accept donations could thereby exploit two classes of donors. They could exploit donors who would donate whether or not compensation was offered but who would prefer to receive compensation. And they could exploit donors who would only donate when they believe that there would be a shortfall in the plasma supply as a result of the prohibition of donor compensation.

Current Commercial Plasma Centers Do Not Exploit Their Donors

It is thus *in theory* possible for plasma donors to be exploited both by plasma centers that offer compensation for donations and by plasma centers that are precluded from doing so by the prohibition of donor compensation. But do either of these types of plasma centers exploit their donors *in practice*?

For a commercial plasma center to exploit its donors it would either have to manipulate the amount of compensation that it offers so that it fails to reflect the relationship between the supply of plasma and the demand for it, where this would work to its benefit, or else benefit from such manipulation by a third party. There is no reason to believe that current commercial plasma centers exploit their donors in either of these ways. Within the United States, no plasma center that compensates its donors has a legal monopoly to operate within a geographic area. They thus do not exploit their donors through using such a monopoly to reduce the level of compensation that they offer below that which would reflect the relationship between the supply of plasma and the demand for it. Instead, they compete with each other for donors. The level of compensation that they offer thus varies according to, for example, the relative demand for plasma, the economic conditions of the area in which they are located, competition from other proximate plasma centers, and whether the center is running any promotions to incentivize donation.

The plasma company Grifols, for example, states clearly that rates of compensation will vary between its different collections centers and that this will depend in part on whether a center is running a promotion. They state that on average plasma donors can expect to receive around $200 a month.[3] They also offer additional rewards through their "Buddy Bonus" referral program.[4] CSL Plasma also states that compensation levels will vary but notes that new donors could receive up to $400 a month. CSL offers new donors in New Jersey a $10 coupon that they can redeem at the CSL location in Hamilton, New Jersey.[5] B Positive Plasma boasts that their New Jersey donors can earn over $500 a month. They also offer additional rewards for referring others who become donors.[6] Octapharma Plasma states that new donors could receive up to $400 a month by donating plasma; they could also be eligible for e-gift cards and sweepstakes promotions if they joined the reward program OPI+ Rewards.[7] That these companies note that compensation will vary by location, differ in the types of secondary incentives that they offer donors, and vary in the amount of compensation that they suggest a first-time donor could receive (while clustering around $400 a month) indicates that they are competing for donors. It is thus likely that the amount of compensation that commercial plasma centers in the United States offer their donors reflects the relationship between the supply of plasma and demand for it. There should thus be a strong presumption in favor of the view that they do not exploit their donors on the account of exploitation developed earlier.

But while commercial plasma centers in the United States operate in a competitive environment that precludes them from exploiting their donors, this is not true of plasma centers in Germany, Austria, and the Czech Republic which offer compensation. In these countries – the three European countries which allow donors to be financially compensated – the levels of compensation that plasma centers can offer are fixed by law.[8] In Germany compensation is set at between 19 and 22 Euros depending on how much plasma is collected (which in turn is also set by law and depends on the donor's weight),[9] while in Austria donors can receive 18 Euros in compensation for donating.[10] In the Czech Republic compensation is limited to c. $20.[11] These compensation levels do not reflect the relationship between the supply of plasma and the demand for it. Instead, they are the result of third-party interference with this price signal. Since this is so the first condition for these plasma centers to exploit their donors has been met. The question of whether they exploit their donors thus turns on whether they benefit from this interference with the price signal.

One might try to determine if this is the case by asking whether the level of compensation that must be legally offered is *higher* or *lower* than that which would be offered were it to function as a price signal in a market setting free from the interference of this price-fixing. Consider a situation where the level of compensation that plasma centers in these countries are legally required to offer is *higher* than that which they would need to offer to secure sufficient plasma to meet demand in a situation in which third-party price-fixing was absent. In this situation, they would not benefit from the third-party interference with the price signals. They would thus not exploit their donors. (In fact, a case could be made that their donors are – possibly blamelessly – exploiting them!)

What of a situation where the level of compensation that the plasma centers in these countries must offer their donors is *lower* than that which they would offer their donors in a market setting? It is tempting to claim that were this to be the case then they would exploit their donors by offering (albeit under duress) a lower rate than they would otherwise need to offer. After all, absent third-party interference with the price signal they would provide their donors with *more* compensation for the *same* donation and so the artificial lowering of the amount of compensation offered would appear to work to their benefit. This tempting line of argument would also provide a pleasing symmetry: If market levels of compensation would be *lower* than that which plasma centers are legally required to offer prospective donors then they would *not* exploit them, while if they were *higher*, then they *would*.

But while it is tempting to hold that plasma centers in these European countries exploit their donors in situations where compensation levels are fixed if absent such fixing the levels of compensation that they would offer would rise this is not the case. It is possible that being required to offer donors a lower level of compensation than would be offered in a competitive market for donors could work to a plasma center's detriment. This would be the case if by increasing the compensation that it offered the plasma center could generate enough profit from the additional donations that it would thus secure to more than offset the additional cost of compensating its donors at the higher level.[12] If this were so, then it would be better off if it was allowed to offer a higher rate of compensation than it is allowed to offer when the rate was fixed by law. To illustrate this, compare two different scenarios. In Scenario 1 a plasma center must legally offer $20 compensation per donation. At this level of compensation, it makes $10 profit per donation. At a compensation level of $20, it secures 1000 donations a week. It thus makes a profit of $10,000 a week. In Scenario 2 it can set its own level of compensation. It recognizes that were it to secure more donations it could make more overall profit even if its profit per donation decreased. It now offers $25 per donation and so makes $5 profit on each one. (The price at which it sells its plasma or plasma-derived products remains unchanged as do its other costs per unit; all that changes is the level of compensation offered for source plasma.) By offering $25 per donation, it secures 2,100 donors a week. It thus makes a profit of $10,500 a week. Fixing the level of competition at $20 thus works to the *detriment* of the plasma center – not to its advantage.[13] A rise in the level of compensation that plasma centers in these European countries would offer prospective donors once mandated compensation levels were removed thus does not indicate that they had benefitted from their interference in the price signal. One would thus not be justified in inferring from the fact that the level of compensation that must legally be offered is *lower* than that which would be offered in a situation free from this interference that the plasma centers subject to it had thereby exploited their donors.

European plasma centers that offer donors financial compensation would thus not benefit from being legally required to offer a level of compensation that is higher than that which they would offer in a market setting in which compensation was not subject to the control of a third party. But they could also fail to benefit from being legally required to offer donors a level of compensation that is lower than that which they would offer in a market setting in which compensation were not subject to the control of a third party. Unless the mandated compensation levels in those European countries that allow plasma centers to financially compensate their donors are identical with the levels of compensation that they would offer absent this constraint (i.e., if bureaucratic fiat happened to hit upon the precise level of compensation that would be offered in a situation where this was determined by the interaction of supply and demand) the imposition of mandated compensation levels will work to their detriment. There is thus good reason to believe that these centers do not benefit from being subject to mandates concerning the levels of compensation that they can offer their donors. There is thus good reason to believe that they do not exploit their donors.

Do Plasma Centers That Are Prohibited From Compensating Their Donors Exploit Them?

There is thus good reason to believe that neither American nor European plasma agencies that offer financial compensation to their donors exploit them. But what of those plasma centers that operate under legal regimes that prohibit donor compensation – do they exploit their donors?

The answer to this question will depend on whether either one of the two classes of donors that were identified previously as being those that could be exploited by plasma centers that are legally prohibited from offering compensation actually donate to them. Recall, the first class of donors that were identified previously as being vulnerable to such exploitation consists of those who would donate whether or not compensation is offered, but who would prefer to receive compensation. The second class of vulnerable donors are those who would only donate if they believed that there will be a shortage of plasma as a result of the prohibition of donor compensation. Determining whether any actual donors fall into these classes is not straightforward. While there are many studies that address the question of what motivates donors to donate there are none that ask those who are not financially compensated for their donations whether they would prefer to be so compensated. Nor are there any studies that ask donors whether they would prefer not to donate but would do so without compensation if they believed that there would be a shortage of plasma if they (and others) did not. There is, however, indirect evidence that both classes of donors do exist.

The First Class of Vulnerable Donors: Those Who Would Donate Whether or Not Compensation Is Offered, but Who Would Prefer to Receive Compensation

In groundbreaking work, Nicola Lacetera and Mario Macis examined the effects that National Law 584 (1967) had on blood donation in Italy.[14] This law gives Italian blood donors the right to a paid day off work on the same day that they donate blood or blood components. It applies to persons who are employees, whether of private or public firms; the salary and contributions that they would receive for the day that they take off are reimbursed by the State.[15] Lacetera's and Macis' analysis was based on a longitudinal dataset that consisted of "the individual histories of blood donations of the whole population of donors in an Italian mid-sized town."[16] This database included information of the c. 2,600 donors' occupations and their labor market status in the periods 1985–1989 and 2002–2006 in addition to their demographic information.[17] Donations could only be made in the morning in the town's hospital, and most employees did not work on Saturday. This means that if an employee wished to maximize the number of consecutive days off that she enjoyed then she should donate on a Friday.[18] A donor who was not an employee – and so who would not benefit from Law 584 – would not be similarly motivated to donate on a Friday. Lacetera's and Macis' longitudinal data enabled them to correlate changes in donors' labor market status (from employee to nonemployee or from nonemployee to employee) with changes in the frequency with which they donated blood. They found that Law 584 induced additional donations from donors who were employees, with "donors who go from being nonemployees to being employees" increasing the frequency with which they donated.[19] From this Lacetera and Macis concluded that Law 584 stimulates more donations from people who are already donors.[20] This finding also supports the claim that some donors who would donate in the absence of compensation would prefer to donate when compensation is offered. Law 584 did not provide any compensation for donors who were nonemployees.

If these donors were indifferent to receiving compensation for their donations, we would expect the number of times they donated to remain the
same when they became employees (and so able to receive compensation
for their donation under Law 584). But this was not the case. Instead, as
Lacetera and Macis note, the number of times that these donors donated
increased once they could receive compensation for them under Law 584.
Thus, while these donors did donate in the absence of compensation,
they were not indifferent to it but preferred to receive it. There thus are
some donors who would donate whether or not compensation is offered
but who would prefer to receive it.

This conclusion can also be drawn from a study conducted by Lacetera, Macis, and Slonim on the effects of incentives on blood donations
to the American Red Cross (ARC) in northern Ohio between May 2006
and October 2008.[21] They found that when incentives were offered "both
the numbers of donors who attempted to donate and the number of units
of blood collected" increased significantly (between 15% and 20%).[22]
Using the cost that the ARC paid for each incentive item as a proxy for
the value that each held for the donor they also found "a positive and
significant relationship between the cost of the incentives and turnout
and units collected."[23] This result was corroborated by evidence from
a natural field experiment that they ran between September 2009 and
August 2010 at 72 ARC blood drives.[24]

These findings do not by themselves necessarily support the claim that
(some) donors who would donate plasma without compensation would
prefer to receive compensation for their donations. This is because they
are consistent with the view that there are two types of donors: "Pure"
pro-social donors (who would donate without compensation but not
when it is offered) and donors who donate only to receive the incentive
on offer. It is possible that the former type of donor left the donor pool
when incentives were offered to be replaced by larger numbers of the second type of donors.[25] But while this is possible it is not the case. Instead,
Lacetera, Macis, and Slomin found that donors shifted their donations
away from blood drives that did not offer incentives toward neighboring
drives (within two miles' drive) occurring at similar times that offered
incentives.[26] In an "average drive" scenario (where the value of the incentive offered was $3) c. 45% of the additional donors that attended would
be donors who would have otherwise donated at a neighboring drive.[27]
This displacement of donors from unincentivized drives to those that
offered incentives increased if the incentives that were being offered were
of a higher monetary value.[28] This supports the claim that some donors
who would donate whether or not compensation is offered would prefer
to receive it.[29]

A defender of prohibition might at this point object, noting that these
studies focused on the donation of blood, not plasma, and that the compensation offered was not financial but either paid time off work or items

such as T-shirts, coupons, sweaters, coolers, or umbrellas.[30] Given these disanalogies, she might continue, this study does not support the claim that there are any *plasma* donors who would donate in the absence of *financial* compensation but who would prefer to receive it.

The first response to this objection is to note that since there are blood donors who would prefer to donate without compensation rather than not donate at all, but who would prefer to donate with compensation rather than without it, it is not unreasonable to believe that there will be some donors of similar body parts (e.g., plasma) that would also have this preference ranking. Thus, while these studies only definitively show that there are *blood* donors with this preference ranking their existence supports the claim that there are also plasma donors with this preference.

The second response to this objection concedes that financial and nonfinancial incentives can affect donors' motivations differently. (This was seen in Mellstrom's and Johannesson's field experiment discussed in Chapter 2, where rewarding a person for donating blood by donating SEK 50 to charity had, for some donors, a more positive effect on their motivation to donate blood than did a direct payment of SEK 50 to them.)[31] It is thus possible that a donor who, for example, preferred to receive a paid day off work for donating, to donating without receiving this benefit would *not* prefer to receive a financial reward for donating to not receiving such a reward. It is also possible that a donor who preferred to receive, for example, a paid day off work for donating, to donating without this benefit would also prefer *not* to receive financial compensation for donating to receiving this in exchange for her donation. To establish that the work of Lacetera and Macis, and Lacetera, Macis, and Slomin support the view that some donors who would donate whether or not compensation is offered would prefer to receive it, it must be shown that the donors referenced in their work would prefer to receive financial compensation to no compensation at all, just as they would prefer to receive, for example, paid days off work or trinkets to no compensation at all. Absent further information about the preferences of the donors referenced in Lacetera, Macis, and Slomin's study it cannot be assumed from the mere fact that they would prefer to receive trinkets for donating rather than to receive no material reward at all that they would similarly prefer to receive financial compensation for donating rather than to receive no material reward at all. (Although given the preferences that they exhibited it is likely that they would have this preference ranking.) The work of Lacetera and Macis, however, *does* establish that some donors would prefer to receive financial compensation for donating rather than no material reward at all, even though they would still donate in the absence of extrinsic incentives. In offering prospective blood donors a paid day off work in exchange for donating, Law 584 *de facto* offers them a choice between being paid to perform their usual job or being paid to donate blood. In donating blood and taking the paid day off (their usual) work in exchange some donors demonstrated that they would prefer to be (*de facto*) paid to donate blood rather than to perform their usual job. Since some of the donors affected by Law 584 donated in the absence of the compensation that it offered them but demonstrated through their actions that they preferred to receive it, then it is the case that there are some donors who would donate in the absence of financial compensation but who would prefer to receive it. The first class of donors that were identified previously as being vulnerable to exploitation by plasma centers that are prohibited from offering compensation (i.e., those who would donate whether or not compensation is offered, but who would prefer to receive compensation) thus exists.

The Second Class of Vulnerable Donors: Those Who Would Only Donate if They Believed That There Will Be a Shortage of Plasma as a Result of the Prohibition of Donor Compensation

Are there any donors who would only donate if they believed that if they (and others) do not, then there will be a shortage of plasma procured owing to the prohibition of donor compensation? Some organizations that procure plasma appear to believe so. For example, to motivate people to donate plasma Canadian Blood Services (CBS) emphasizes that there is a "looming threat to the supply of plasma needed to produce plasma protein products for Canadian patients today and in the future."[32] In response to this "threat" to Canadian patients CBS "intends to significantly increase plasma collections" within their "voluntary, unpaid system."[33] The approach that they are taking is clear: Believing that some donors would only donate if they thought that there would be a shortage of plasma relative to demand CBS is publicizing this shortage. Their emphasis on the "unpaid" nature of their procurement system could be read as an implicit acknowledgment that the shortages they are experiencing are owed to the prohibition of donor compensation, and an appeal to those donors for whom this origin of the shortage matters. A similar approach is being taken in France. The Etablissement Francais du Sang (EFS) currently emphasizes how "rare and precious" plasma from persons with AB blood type is and how (together with donors with blood type B) "sought after" such donors are.[34] The message that there is a shortage of plasma from people with certain blood types was reinforced by EFS from January 6 to January 18, 2020 with their "Missing Type" campaign. This campaign – featured throughout the EFS website and on social media – removed the letters of the most-needed blood types from the website's prose to emphasize that these were "missing" from inventory.[35] In both the CBS campaign and the EFS campaign the message is clear: Plasma donations are needed to offset the current shortages. And since neither CBS nor EFS offer financial compensation to their donors their propagation of this message indicates that they believe that some donors will only donate without compensation if they believe that their donations are needed to offset the shortage that would otherwise occur.

But this indicates only that some organizations that procure plasma *believe* that there is a class of donors that would only donate in a situation where they believed that their donations were needed to offset shortfalls that resulted from the prohibition of compensation. It does not show that such donors *actually* exist. But while there have been no studies specifically conducted to determine if there are any such donors there is evidence of their existence. Recognizing the increased demand for plasma-derived products within Australia, Bove et al. conducted a study to determine what triggered donors' initial (financially uncompensated) plasma donation and what factors were associated with continued donation.[36] While they discovered that the main trigger for an initial donation was a personal request from a collection center's staff member they also noted that "some donors expressed an obligation to donate, because they were aware of the medical need for plasma products, but believed that few people participate in plasmapheresis."[37] This provides evidence that the organizations that procure plasma from uncompensated donors are justified in believing that some donors will only donate without compensation if they believe that their donations are needed to offset the shortage that would otherwise occur in a system where compensation is prohibited.

Donor Exploitation

There is, then, evidence that both classes of donors that are vulnerable to exploitation by plasma centers that do not compensate their donors exist. If any of these donors have donated to plasma centers that are prohibited from compensating them for their donations then, on the analysis of exploitation developed in the last chapter and explicated earlier, these centers would have exploited them. Since it is highly likely that some donors who would donate without compensation but would prefer to receive it will have donated to plasma centers that are prohibited from compensating them it is highly likely that some donors have been exploited by the (non-compensating) plasma centers to which they donated. Similarly, it is also highly likely that some donors who would only donate in situations where they believed that their donations were needed to offset shortfalls that result from the prohibition of donor compensation will also have donated to plasma centers that are prohibited from offering them compensation. (Indeed, both CBS and EFS have *encouraged* this.) These donors would thus also have been exploited by the centers to which they donated.

That some donors are exploited by the plasma centers to which they donate but which are prohibited from compensating them for their donations does not entail that such centers exploit *all* of their donors. Donors that would donate only in the absence of compensation to secure third-party recognition of their pro-social attitudes will not be exploited. These donors do not have a relationship with the plasma centers for which the question of whether one party has gained at the expense of the other could arise. This question is only pertinent to transactional relationships in which each party incurs costs and receives from the other benefits in return. This is not the type of relationship that these donors have with the plasma centers. Instead, their relationship with them is one in which the centers provide them with the opportunity to secure something that they value (i.e., social approval) from third parties. These donors are thus not exploited by the plasma centers to which they donate their plasma. And donors who would be indifferent to any offered compensation would similarly fail to be in a transactional relationship with the procurement agencies. They would thus be invulnerable to exploitation by the plasma centers that are prohibited from offering them compensation.

Sauce for the Goose, Sauce for the Gander

We have now reached a surprising conclusion. The surprise is not that commercial plasma centers do not exploit their donors. While the earlier arguments show that the common complaint that compensated donors are exploited by commercial plasma centers is mistaken it is not that surprising – especially given the paucity of argument that offered in support of this objection by those who propose it. What *is* surprising is that prohibiting donor compensation leads to the exploitation of two classes of donors by those plasma centers that are prohibited from offering donor compensation. These donors are those who would prefer to receive compensation but do not, and those who only donate because they believe that there is a shortage of plasma available relative to demand owing to the prohibition of donor compensation. Rather than donor exploitation occurring when donor compensation is legally permitted it actually occurs when donor compensation is legally prohibited. Those concerned with avoiding donor compensation (as all should be) should thus support allowing compensation rather than supporting its prohibition.

This conclusion is so surprising that one might suspect that it has been arrived at by sleight of hand. In particular, one might worry that it is merely an artifact of the account of exploitation that was developed in the previous chapter. But it is not. Before showing why I should address an immediate objection that might be raised to the aforementioned argument for the conclusion that plasma centers that are prohibited from compensating their donors thereby exploit some of them.

In my discussion of the commercial plasma centers that operate in Europe, I argued that even if the level of compensation that they would offer their donors were they not bound by the amounts set by the State would rise one could not infer from this that they were benefitting from being required to offer lower levels of compensation than they otherwise would do. However, when discussing the possibly exploitative practice of plasma centers that were prohibited from offering compensation to their donors, I argued that we could infer from the fact that they offered $0 to their donors when, absent this price ceiling they would need to offer more, that they were benefitting from this price ceiling. These claims appear to be in tension. How can I consistently hold that commercial plasma centers do *not* benefit from price ceilings while also holding that their noncommercial counterparts *do* benefit from them?

The answer to this question lies in the nature of the benefits that these different types of plasma centers pursue. The commercial plasma centers (primarily) pursue profit.[38] Given this, capping the level of compensation that they can offer could (as I outlined earlier) work to their detriment by reducing their profitability. By contrast, noncommercial plasma centers (e.g., those that are run "not for profit" and that operate in situations where donor compensation is prohibited) are not concerned with maximizing their profitability. The benefits that they receive from obtaining plasma lie elsewhere. It might be tempting to claim that they benefit from helping the patients that require PDMPs. But while they no doubt aim at this – as do commercial plasma centers – this cannot be their primary goal. If it were then given the empirical evidence (outlined in Chapter 1) that shows how effective donor compensation is in securing plasma, then they would be actively lobbying to be freed from the shackles of its prohibition. But they do not do so. Since this is so, even without identifying the benefit that they are pursuing it is reasonable to infer that the price ceiling (of $0) that is imposed upon them does not work substantially to their detriment. It is also reasonable to infer that it works to their *advantage*. The primary benefit pursued by plasma centers that operate in situations where donor compensation is prohibited is clearly not connected to maximizing the amount of plasma that they procure. (If it were, again, they would lobby to be freed from the price cap of $0.) It is also not connected to maximizing their revenues. (They are, after all, noncommercial entities.) But even without identifying the primary goal of such centers, it is reasonable to assume that they benefit from minimizing their expenditures in pursuit of it.[39] As noted earlier, this would be achieved by securing plasma from donors who would donate whether or not they were offered compensation but who would prefer to receive it rather than not. It would also be achieved by securing plasma without compensation from donors who would only donate as they believed that the amount of plasma being procured was falling short of that required to satisfy patient needs as a result of the prohibition of donor compensation. Thus, while it is reasonable to infer from their actions that commercial plasma centers are adversely affected by caps being placed in the amount of compensation that they can offer it is also reasonable to infer from their actions that plasma centers that operate in situations where compensation is prohibited are not similarly adversely affected. The apparent tension between the claim that commercial plasma centers do *not* benefit from price ceilings and the claim that their noncommercial counterparts *do* benefit is thus resolved.

Stacking the Deck? Donor Compensation and Alternative Analyses of Exploitation

I noted earlier that the conclusion that prohibiting donor compensation results in the exploitation of two classes of donors by plasma centers that operate under such prohibitive regimes is so surprising that one might suspect that it is merely an artifact of the account of exploitation that was developed in the previous chapter.

To allay this suspicion, I will consider how plasma centers that compensate their donors and those that are prohibited from doing so fare when their treatment of their donors is assessed against two alternative accounts of exploitation. The first of these is a neo-Lockean model of exploitation that assesses whether C exploited X by reference to the prices that would be paid for the goods and services they exchange in a hypothetical market.[40] The second is a very different account of exploitation which will serve well to allay the fears of those concerned about market-orientated analyses: The Marxian account of exploitation developed by Paul Hughes.[41]

Neo-Lockean Exploitation

The first alternative account of exploitation that I will consider assesses whether C exploited X by comparing the price of the good or service exchanged in their transaction with its hypothetical market price. On this neo-Lockean account of exploitation, C exploited X when the price that he charged her (or that he paid to her) differs from that which he would have received (or paid) were a competitive market for the good or service in question to exist. (C would exploit X were this price differential work to her favor in the actual transaction.)[42] For example, were A the only owner of a tug available to save ship B from wrecking by drifting into ship C he would exploit the owners of B if he offered to tow her to safety for $10,000 when he would only be able to charge them $500 were there other tugs available to compete with him.[43]

Given that this is still a market-oriented account of exploitation it would in many cases provide an answer to the question of whether C exploited X that would be the same as that provided by the analysis of exploitation that I outlined and defended in the previous chapter. And it might still allow C to charge X extremely high rates in certain rescue situations, such as that of Situation 4. However, it might seem that on this analysis of exploitation plasma centers that do not compensate their donors as they were prohibited from doing so would *not* be guilty of exploiting those donors who would only donate when they believe that there will be a shortage of plasma relative to demand owing to the prohibition of donor compensation. The reason for this is simple. On this analysis of exploitation to assess if (actual) donors were exploited the amount of compensation that they (actually) received for their donations will be compared to that which they would have received for them in a (hypothetical) market where plasma was a commodified good at all stages of its supply chain. This hypothetical market mirrors in all respects the actual market that would exist were plasma commodified in this way. But since this is so the plasma that is procured in this hypothetical market would only be procured from those donors who would donate in a situation where compensation for their donations was offered. Donors who would only donate plasma when they believed that there would be a shortage of it relative to demand would not donate were it to be procured by market means. In the situation of the hypothetical market, they would believe that donor compensation would secure the amount of plasma needed. They would thus believe that there would be no need for them to donate to attempt to make up a shortfall. These donors would thus receive $0 for their plasma. A plasma center that (actually) secured plasma from them in the situation when they would (actually) donate (i.e., one where compensation was prohibited) would thus provide them with the same amount of compensation that they would receive in a hypothetical market (i.e., $0). Thus, on this neo-Lockean account of exploitation, the (actual) plasma centers that secured plasma from this class of donors without compensating them for it would not have exploited them.

While this argument is superficially plausible it has gone badly awry.[44] I will uncover where it goes wrong shortly. But before I do so I should make two initial observations about the use of a neo-Lockean analysis of exploitation to defend the prohibition of donor compensation from the charge that this will lead to the exploitation of certain classes of donors. First, those who adopt a neo-Lockean account of exploitation must concede that compensating donors at the actual market rate cannot exploit them. This entails that only policies governing the procurement of, for example, plasma that depart from this (e.g., the prohibition of donor compensation) could exploit donors. Adopting a neo-Lockean account of exploitation thus places the opponent of donor compensation on the defensive. Offers of donor compensation are not exploitative on this view if they are made within a competitive marketplace. However, on this view, the prohibition of donor compensation is not similarly automatically nonexploitative. The opponent of donor compensation (but not its defender) is thus vulnerable to the charge that her preferred approach to plasma procurement will exploit donors. Second, adopting a neo-Lockean analysis of exploitation would still lead to the conclusion that donors who would donate even if compensation were not offered but who would prefer to receive it, would be exploited by plasma centers that operated when compensation was prohibited and so did not compensate their donors. In a hypothetical market, these donors would have received compensation for their donations. They would thus have been exploited by the non-compensating plasma centers to the degree that this hypothetical compensation differs from $0. Adopting a neo-Lockean analysis of exploitation can thus only attempt to limit the scope of the donor exploitation that non-compensating plasma centers engage in when compensation is prohibited. It does not absolve them of this charge entirely.

It is now time to explain why the aforementioned neo-Lockean defense of non-compensating plasma centers against the charge that they exploit those donors who would only donate plasma when they believe that there would be a shortfall as a result of the prohibition of donor compensation goes awry. That argument focused on how much these donors would have received had there been a market for plasma. It then determines that they would not have received any compensation as they would not have donated in such a market. From this, it concludes that such donors are not exploited when compensation is prohibited on the grounds that in this situation, they would have received the same amount for their plasma ($0) as they would have received in the hypothetical market (i.e., when they did not donate). But this misses the point of using a neo-Lockean analysis of exploitation morally to assess a transaction. This analysis of exploitation can only assess the morality of those actual transactions that have hypothetical counterparts. If the transaction would not have taken place in the hypothetical situation, then this analysis of exploitation cannot be used to assess the morality of the actual transaction that occurred. This neo-Lockean analysis of exploitation thus cannot establish that donors who would only donate in a situation where compensation is prohibited because they believe that their donations are needed to help rectify the shortage of plasma would not be exploited by the non-compensating plasma centers that take their donations. Owing to the absence of a hypothetical market to price their donations this analysis of exploitation must remain silent on the question of whether or not they were *actually* exploited. This account of exploitation thus cannot support the conclusion that such donors were not exploited by the plasma centers to which they donated when donor compensation was prohibited.

Marxian Exploitation

At this point, an opponent of donor compensation might observe that it is not surprising that the neo-Lockean account of exploitation failed to absolve those plasma centers that failed to compensate their donors owing to the prohibition on donor compensation from the charge that they exploited some of them. After all, she might note, this account of exploitation is (like that developed in the previous chapter) still a *market-based* analysis of exploitation. It is thus not surprising that it would condemn anti-market approaches to plasma procurement. Indeed, such an opponent of donor compensation might claim, to assess the conclusions concerning donor compensation that were based on the analysis of exploitation in the last chapter by way of an analysis of exploitation that was based on a hypothetical market is not really to offer an independent assessment at all. It is, instead, akin to checking the political claim expressed in one newspaper against those made in another that was owned by the same tycoon.[45]

These are fair points. But the concerns of even this opponent of donor compensation can be allayed by assessing the aforementioned claims concerning donor compensation and exploitation against a nonmarket, *Marxian* analysis of exploitation: That developed by Paul Hughes.

There are two reasons to choose Hughes' account of exploitation to demonstrate that the surprising conclusions of this chapter are not merely a function of the account of exploitation developed in the last. First, as a Marxian account, it is clearly not predisposed to look favorably upon commercial plasma centers and askance at those that rely on uncompensated donation. (Indeed, Marx's famous dictum "from each according to his ability, to each according to his need" indicates that if anything any slant in a Marxian account of exploitation would be in favor of the latter type of center rather than the former.)[46] Second, Hughes developed his Marxian account of exploitation in response to Gerald Dworkin's argument for legalizing a market in kidneys. Given this origin, this account of exploitation is relevant to the related question of whether plasma centers exploit their donors.[47]

Hughes begins his account of exploitation by stating that

> [e]xploitation is not just what happens when a worker labors in a factory for a wage, it's what happens *to make that happen.* In other words, exploitation involves the background set of options which impel worker's [sic] to "choose" to labor for capitalists.[48]

Persons who are exploited are, writes Hughes, "in political and economic circumstances that enable them to be used to benefit others not in such restrictive circumstances."[49] Their exploiters are "using" them not merely because they are "underpaid and overworked" but because "the reasonable alternatives available to them are so limited that the addition of certain kinds of options may have a debilitating impact on a person's autonomy and well-being."[50] A person who is concerned with the moral value of autonomy or well-being should thus object to the introduction of certain options into persons' choice sets: Those that would "presuppose and/or [if chosen] reinforce the status quo."[51] Hughes concludes from this Marxian account of exploitation that a market in kidneys should not be allowed. Such a market would presuppose that there were poor people whose economic situation would lead them to sell an organ. It would also reinforce the status quo, possibly by further physically debilitating the sellers so that their opportunities for employment would be even more limited than they were prior to the sale.[52] It could thus be expected to reduce both the value of their autonomy and their well-being.[53] The former could be compromised as a result of the physical effects of the sale further restricting the number of viable choices they have after it. (Their post-sale ability to perform manual labor, for example, will be limited.) The latter could be compromised both by the physical effects of the sale and by subjecting them to "psychic distress" at the prospect of the "necessary evil" of selling a kidney.[54]

Unfortunately for the opponents of donor compensation, both classes of donors that were identified as being exploited by plasma centers that accepted their donations in situations where compensation was prohibited will still be exploited by them on this Marxian account of exploitation.

Hughes begins his Marxian account of exploitation by noting that the background conditions against which the potentially exploitative transaction takes place are relevant to determining if exploitation has occurred. The background conditions that are relevant to assessing whether the introduction of the option to donate plasma where compensation for such donation is prohibited is exploitative include the fact that there is an unmet medical need for plasma. They also include the fact that the previously mentioned two classes of potential donors exist: Those that would donate were compensation not to be offered but who would prefer that it was, and those who would only donate when they believe that this is needed to help rectify the shortage of plasma generated by the prohibition of donor compensation.

Against these background conditions, the introduction of the option to donate plasma will, when combined with the prohibition of compensated donation, enable the plasma centers that offer it to use both of these vulnerable classes of donors for their own benefit. They will be able to secure plasma from them without the need to compensate them. And they will be able to do this because offering only the option to donate plasma without the option to receive compensation for this will limit the alternatives available to them so that they can only "choose" to donate without compensation.[55] The introduction of this option thus meets Hughes' initial condition for it to be an option whose introduction into a person's choice set could lead to her exploitation. Just as (on Hughes' Marxian account) capitalist exploitation involves the background set of options that impel workers to "choose" to work for capitalists so too does the exploitation of certain classes of donors involve background conditions that impel them to "choose" to donate to plasma centers without compensation.

The introduction of the option to donate without compensation against the background conditions outlined earlier would also reinforce the status quo. The donors who would donate but would prefer to be compensated for doing so would continue to donate although their desire for compensation continues to be thwarted. Owing to the prohibition of compensation and the consequent shortfall in the amount of plasma collected domestically the donors who would only donate when they believed that this was needed to make up such shortfalls would also continue to donate. In this way, the status quo is perpetuated.

Finally, limiting these donors' options in this way will have an adverse effect on their well-being when compared with the alternative situation in which they have the option to donate where compensation for such donation is allowed (but not required). The first class of donors would be better off in this alternative situation as they would prefer to receive compensation for their donation. The second class of donors would also be better off in this alternative situation as they would be justified in believing that the amount of plasma that would be secured through compensated donation would meet medical needs – and this would release them from the obligation to donate to make up any shortfall from this. On Hughes' Marxian account of exploitation, then, the introduction of the option to donate plasma where compensation for such donation is prohibited would be exploitative of those members of these two classes of donors who chose to pursue it.

However, there would not necessarily be any such exploitation in a regime that allowed compensated donation. This might seem surprising since Hughes' account of exploitation was developed to respond to an argument in favor of compensating the donors of human body parts. But Hughes' aim was to argue against compensating *kidney* donors, not *plasma* donors. Since his argument rests on empirical claims concerning the effects of compensation and since nephrectomy is far more involved and dangerous than plasmapheresis it is possible that it could be sound against markets in kidneys but inapplicable to the offer of compensation to plasma donors.[56]

The existence of commercial plasma centers would presuppose the existence of persons who would be willing to donate for compensation, just as the existence of commercial firms of kidney buyers would presuppose the existence of persons willing to sell them. But while an explanation of how a kidney market might reinforce the economic impoverishment of compensated kidney donors is available (it will compromise the health of donors so that they would have fewer employment opportunities post-sale) no such explanation is forthcoming to establish that allowing donor compensation would reinforce the economic status of plasma donors.[57] This is important. On Hughes' Marxian account of exploitation, the introduction of an option into a person's choice set could lead to her exploitation if (a) it presupposed that the background against which it was introduced was one where she had limited viable options, and (b) her pursuit of this option would reinforce her position as someone with limited options. But while (a) might hold in the context of commercial plasma procurement (b) does not.

Unlike the removal of a kidney, plasmapheresis is unlikely to adversely affect a donor's ability to work. Moreover, the amount of money that is typically offered to plasma donors is too small for them to become economically dependent upon it. The typical plasma donor in the United States is compensated $35 for each donation and donates fifteen times; she thus receives $525 a year.[58] Even the most motivated donor in the United States who donated the maximum of 104 times a year would receive a comparatively small amount of $3,600 annually.[59] (These figures should be striking to everyone familiar with Titmuss' work. In *The Gift Relationship*, he claimed that "[s]ome plasmapheresis donors, double bled twice a week, received $6,240 per month in fees in 1968."[60] In 2021 dollars $6,240 is c. $49,340. According to the figure cited by Titmuss – and assuming that a donor would donate twice a week for a four-week month, or 8 times in total – the claim is that plasma donors were receiving c. $6,168 in 2021 dollars per donation. This is utterly implausible – especially when Titmuss earlier claimed that "[s]ome regular [plasma] donors are, in effect, 'semi-salaried' and paid $150–200 a month for a specified number of donations" – an amount that Titmuss considered to be "high."[61] As far as I know I am the first to notice this oddity in Titmuss' data.[62]) And there is evidence that even though compensation encourages repeat donation of blood and blood products it does not typically lead to a long-term commitment.[63] (Donors in the United States, for example, typically only donate for six months.)[64] Thus, while the existence of a commercial system of plasma procurement might presuppose the existence of prospective donors it would not reinforce the economic status quo.[65] Donors neither become economically dependent upon it nor does their participation as donors adversely affect either the number or quality of their economic options either during their tenure as donors or after this. Hughes' Marxian account of exploitation thus does not support the claim that offering compensation to plasma donors will thereby exploit them.

Which Analysis of Exploitation Should We Accept?

The conclusion that from the point of view of one concerned with avoiding exploitation regimes that allow donor compensation are morally preferable to regimes that prohibit this is thus not merely an artifact of the account of exploitation that was developed in the last chapter.[66]

But it was important for this conclusion to be established on the basis of that account of exploitation rather than on the basis of either the neo-Lockean account or Hughes' Marxian accounts. This is because that analysis of exploitation is theoretically superior to both the neo-Lockean account and Hughes' Marxian account. Recall the previous discussion of the claim that the neo-Lockean analysis of exploitation would absolve plasma centers that did not compensate their donors as they were prohibited from doing so from the charge that they exploited the second class of donors. (Those donors who would only donate when compensated were prohibited as they believed that they would then be obligated to make up the shortfall that would result.) I noted there that the neo-Lockean analysis of exploitation was silent on the question of whether or not these donors were exploited. The ability of the neo-Lockean analysis to identify when a transaction is exploitative is thus more limited than that of the analysis of exploitation developed in the previous chapter. Since that account of exploitation is thus more theoretically complete than its neo-Lockean rival its adoption is theoretically preferable.

The account of exploitation that was developed in the previous chapter is also more theoretically satisfying than Hughes'. This is because it is broader. Hughes' account of exploitation cannot, for example, accommodate the (plausible) view that C exploits both the stranded motorist in Situation 5 and the bartender in Situation 6. The account of exploitation developed in the previous chapter can both accommodate these views and also explain why it is that C's acts are exploitative. Discussion of both the neo-Lockean account of exploitation and Hughes' Marxian account is important to allay any concern that the surprising conclusions of this chapter are merely a product of the account of exploitation developed in the last. But since these analyses of exploitation are theoretically weaker than the account of exploitation developed in the previous chapter, they should not be substituted for it.

Blame and Exploitation

In this chapter, I have established that some donors are exploited by plasma centers in situations where donor compensation is prohibited. But that leaves open the question of whether plasma centers that operate in those situations are morally blameworthy for this exploitation. As I noted in the previous chapter it is possible for there to be blameless exploitation. Drawing from the variation on Situation 6 ("The Stranger in the Bar") for an exploiter to be blameless for the exploitation that she perpetrates she must be (non-culpably) ignorant that she is engaged in exploitation. She must either be unaware that she is receiving a greater benefit from the transaction than she would have received had there been no agential interference with the price signal, or, if she is aware that she is the beneficiary of such interference, then she must reasonably believe that it has been perpetrated by her trading partner for his own (eventual) benefit. Since The Stranger in the Bar would be aware that drinks are not given away free, it would be implausible for him to claim that he was unaware of any agential interference in the price signal. However, he could claim that he believed that the barman was giving away drinks of his own accord (perhaps as a way to promote the bar). If the Stranger genuinely believed this then (given the other elements of the situation of which he was unaware) he would be blameless for his exploitation of the barman.

Are plasma centers that operate in situations that prohibit donor compensation blameless for the exploitation of (some of) their donors? That depends both on the beliefs that the persons who operate them have and, if their relevant beliefs are false, whether these persons are culpable for having these false beliefs. Like the Stranger in the Bar persons who operate plasma centers in situations where compensation is prohibited cannot (plausibly) claim that they are unaware of any interference with the price signal concerning the relationship between the supply of plasma and the demand for it. Given this, to be blameless for the exploitation of (some of) their donors they must be able to truthfully state that they believed that their donors would not lose anything through donating their plasma without compensation in comparison to a situation in which compensation was offered. This claim would only be true if they believed that *none* of their donors would fall into either of the two vulnerable classes of donors identified earlier.

It is implausible to hold that persons who operate plasma centers in situations where donor compensation is prohibited believe that *none* of their donors would prefer to receive compensation rather than not if this were offered to them. It is hence plausible that their exploitation of these donors is thus blameworthy. There is also reason to believe that the operators of such plasma centers *do* believe that some of their donors are members of the second class of vulnerable donors identified earlier. (Those donors who would prefer not to donate but do so because they believe that there is a shortage of plasma owing to the absence of donor compensation.) Indeed, as I noted earlier, many organizations that procure plasma (such as CBS and EFS) attempt to motivate donation by appealing to the need to combat the shortages of plasma that they are faced with. This indicates that they both know that donors of the second vulnerable class exist and that they wish them to donate. Thus, not only do these organizations exploit these donors – their exploitation of them is blameworthy.

Conclusion

It is widely held that some plasma donors are exploited by the plasma centers to which they donate. This view is correct. Given current practices, some plasma centers *do* exploit some of their donors. But the culprits are not the commercial plasma centers that are the usual target of this criticism. Neither those in the United States nor those in Europe exploit their donors as these centers currently operate. Instead, the exploitative centers are those that operate in legal regimes that *prohibit* the financial compensation of donors. And not only do they exploit some of their donors, but they are *blameworthy* for this exploitation.

But all is not lost for those who oppose donor compensation. They could still argue that (exploitation notwithstanding) a moral concern for social cohesion would justify the prohibition of donor compensation. This approach to defending the prohibition of donor compensation could also be used to solve a puzzle in the debate over donor compensation that is often overlooked: Why is that many countries that prohibit donor compensation within their own borders on the grounds that this is unethical are nonetheless willing to import plasma and PDMPs from other countries that they know procure plasma from compensated donors? I turn to these issues in the next two chapters.

Notes

1. One might object to this claim on the grounds that if the prohibition on compensation was removed then the plasma center could continue to offer $0 to its donors in the expectation that they would continue to donate without compensation. In response, it could be noted that this plasma center might believe that were donors to be aware that compensation was allowed they would refrain from donating without it, even though they would donate when it was prohibited. The center might, for example, believe that when compensation was prohibited, the donors believed that it would compensate them were it allowed to do so, and so view it positively, with this motivating them to donate. It might thus believe that were it not to offer compensation when the ban on this was removed it would lose donations as its donors' view of it changed. It thus offers compensation when the ban is removed. In any case, the purpose of the aforementioned example is simply to show that it is possible for a plasma center that does not compensate its donors to exploit them.
2. The donors will benefit from the satisfaction of having done what they perceive to be their moral duty in a situation where the amount of plasma procured is likely to fall short of that which is needed.
3. See Grifols, "How to Donate Plasma," Available at: www.grifolsplasma.com/en/plasma-donor/how-to-donate/donation-fees
4. See Grifols, "Buddy Bonus Program," Available at: www.grifolsplasma.com/en/returning-plasma-donors/buddy-bonus-program
5. See CSL Plasma, "Coupon Offer," Available at: www.cslplasma.com/center/NJ/199-hamilton/coupon?gclid=EAIaIQobChMIg8WZ9Zn55gIVCaGzCh2-zgwAEAMYASAAEgL4v_D_BwE
6. See B-Positive, "Donate Plasma, Get Paid, Save Lives," Available at: www.bpositivetoday.com/
7. See Octapharma Plasma, "Payments and Rewards," Available at: https://octapharmaplasma.com/donor/payment-rewards
8. The legal status of compensation in Hungary is unclear.
9. European Commission Directorate-General for Health and Food Safety, "Summary Minutes of a Meeting between CSL, PPTA, and DG SANTE P4," (January 21, 2016). Available at: https://ec.europa.eu/health/sites/health/files/blood_tissues_organs/docs/ares20166855155_summary_minutes.pdf
10. Michael Trimmelm, Helene Lattacher, and Monika Janda, "Voluntary Whole-Blood Donors, and Compensated Platelet Donors and Plasma

Donors: Motivation to Donate, Altruism and Aggression," *Transfusion and Apheresis Science* 33 (2005), 149.

11. World Health Organization, *2016 Global Status Report on Blood Safety and* (Geneva: WHO, 2017), 82, note 28.

12. This point is implicit in the observation made by Albert Farrugia, Joshua Penrod, and Jan M. Bult that "commercial interests would not be compensating donors unless it was recognized that this was essential in order to acquire the large volumes of plasma necessary for manufacture." Albert Farrugia, Joshua Penrod, and Jan M. Bult, "The Ethics of Paid Plasma Donation: A Plea for Patient Centeredness," *HEC Forum* 27 (2015), 426.

13. Note that this reinforces the point made in Chapter 2: That imposing a price cap of $0 on donor compensation could be rejected by both donors and plasma centers.

14. Nicola Lacetera and Mario Macis, "Time for Blood: The Effect of Paid Leave Legislation on Altruistic Behavior," *The Journal of Law, Economics, and Organization* 29, 6 (2013), 1384–1420.

15. Ibid., 1385.

16. Ibid., 1387.

17. Ibid.

18. Ibid., 1388.

19. Ibid., 1407–1408.

20. Ibid., 1408–1409. They are careful to note that their data does not support the stronger conclusion that this Law encourages more people to become donors.

21. Nicola Lacetera, Mario Macis, and Robert Slonim, "Will There be Blood? Incentives and Displacement Effects in Pro-Social Behavior," *American Economic Journal* 4, 1 (2012), 186–223.

22. Ibid., 188.

23. Ibid.; the data supporting these claims is outlined on 201–205. This study controlled for differences between the location of the blood drives observed, their hosts, and the degree to which drives with incentives were publicized compared to those where incentives were not offered ensuring that the results were not driven by an unobserved heterogeneity across different locations, hosts, or publicity efforts.

24. Ibid., 189.

25. This possibility will be discussed further in Chapters 6 and 7.

26. Lacetera et al., "Will There be Blood?" 189.

27. Ibid.

28. Ibid.

29. See also Chapter 6, note 48.

30. Lacetera et al., "Will There be Blood?" 194.

31. Mellstrom and Johannesson, "Crowding Out in Blood Donation," 852.

32. See Canadian Blood Services, "Our Commitment to Increasing Plasma Sufficiency in Canada," Available at: https://blood.ca/en/about-us/media/plasma/plasma-sufficiency

33. Ibid.

34. See l'Etablissement français du sang, "Le don de plasma," Available at: https://dondesang.efs.sante.fr/le-don-de-plasma.

35. See l'Etablissement français du sang, "Missing Type," Available at: https://missingtype.efs.sante.fr/.

36. Liliana L. Bove, Tim Bednall, Barbara Masser, and Mark Buzza, "Understanding the Plasmapheresis Donor in a Voluntary, Nonremunerated Environment," *Transfusion* 51 (2011), 2411–2424.

37. Ibid., 2411, 2414.

38. Primarily, but not exclusively. It would be astonishing if they were not also pursuing patient health for its own sake rather than merely as a means to profit.

39. It appears that the primary benefits pursued by some such centers are intended to accrue to their employees. See Taylor, "The Ethics and Politics of Blood Plasma Donation."

40. This account of exploitation is similar to that developed by John Locke in his account of when a price is just. See John Locke, "Venditio," in Mark Goldie, ed., *Locke: Political Essays* (Cambridge: Cambridge University Press, 1999), 339–343.

41. Paul Hughes, "Exploitation, Autonomy, and the Case for Organ Sales," *International Journal of Applied Philosophy* 12, 1 (1998), 89–95.

42. Kenneth J. Arrow gestures toward this account of exploitation in his discussion of Titmuss', *The Gift Relationship*; Kenneth J. Arrow, "Gifts and Exchanges," *Philosophy & Public Affairs* 1, 4 (1972), 357.

43. This example is similar to that of the *Anna* and the *Port Caledonia* that Wertheimer discusses at length; see Wertheimer, *Exploitation*, 40. However, Wertheimer gets the facts of the case wrong; it was not the vessel *Anna* that charged the drifting *Port Caledonia* an "unjust" price to tow her to safety but the tug *Sarah Jolliffe* (which towed the *Port Caledonia* away from the *Anna* so that they would not collide). See Wertheimer, *Exploitation*, 69, and Butler Aspinall, ed., *Reports of Cases Relating to Maritime Law Containing All the Decisions of The Courts of Law and Equity in The United Kingdom* (London, Horace Cox, 1905, vol. 9), 479–480.

44. Indeed, the reasoning here is similar to that of the White Queen in Chapter 5 of Lewis Carroll's, *Through the Looking-Glass, and What Alice Found There* (London: Macmillan & Co., 1872): " 'For instance, now,' she went on, sticking a large piece of plaster on her finger as she spoke, 'there's the King's Messenger. He's in prison now, being punished: and the trial doesn't even begin till next Wednesday: and of course the crime comes last of all.'/'Suppose he never commits the crime?' said Alice./'That would be all the better, wouldn't it?' the Queen said, as she bound the plaster round her finger with a bit of ribbon./Alice felt there was no denying *that*."

45. I thank Jeppe von Platz for pressing me on this point – and doing so in a way that was far more polite than that of this hypothetical opponent of donor compensation!

46. Karl Marx, *The Gotha Program* (New York: National Executive Committee Socialist Labor Party, 1922), 31.

47. Dworkin, "Markets and Morals," 155–161.

48. Hughes, "Exploitation, Autonomy, and the Case for Organ Sales," 92.

49. Ibid.

50. Ibid.

51. Ibid., 93.

52. See the discussion of Hughes' argument in the context of the black market in kidneys in India in Taylor, *Stakes and Kidneys*, 77–80.

53. The relationship between the value of a person's autonomy and her well-being is outlined in Taylor, *Practical Autonomy and Bioethics*, Chapter 10. Note that this is a gloss on Hughes, who holds that the autonomy of those exploited would be compromised.

54. Hughes, "Exploitation, Autonomy, and the Case for Organ Sales," 93.

55. The quotation marks around "choose" are Hughes'.

56. The former is not the case; see Taylor, *Stakes and Kidneys*, 75–80. For a further discussion of the differences between a market in kidneys and

the offer of compensation for plasma donation see the Conclusion of this volume.

57. This way of framing the issue presupposes that compensated plasma donors will be economically similar to compensated kidney donors. But given the differing burdens and compensation levels associated with kidney and plasma donation, there is no reason to believe this.

58. Skinner et al., "Risk-Based Decision Making and Ethical Considerations in Donor Compensation for Plasma-Derived Medicinal Products," 2891. (Note that this claim is compatible with the reported average of 17.5 donations made in 2012 at the 7 plasma centers whose donations were studied by Schreiber and Kimber; it is also compatible with the higher number of donations reported by Bechtloff et al. See Chapter 1, notes 82 and 92.) Given the time involved in making a plasma donation the compensation that donors receive is in line with prevailing wage market wage rates. See J. Mercier Ythier, "The Contested Market of Plasma," 53.

59. Skinner et al., "Risk-Based Decision Making and Ethical Considerations in Donor Compensation for Plasma-Derived Medicinal Products," 2891.

60. Titmuss, *The Gift Relationship*, 77, note 3. Titmuss cites a "personal communication" from Travenol Laboratories International in Morton Grove, Illinois, as the source of this figure.

61. Ibid., 51. A figure of $200 a month for twice-weekly plasma donation can also be extrapolated from Staff author, "Blood Money," *Medical World News* (March 15, 1963), 136.

62. It is possible that Titmuss intended to state that the plasma center in question paid $6, 240 *in total* each month to all of their plasma donors. But this figure would not make sense either, as it would entail that they only had c. 31 donors a month. While the amount of compensation Titmuss cites is implausibly high this number of donors is implausibly low.

63. Christian Weidmanna et al., "Monetary Compensation and Blood Donor Return: Results of a Donor Survey in Southwest Germany," *Transfusion Medicine and Hemotherapy* 41 (2014), 257–262. This survey addressed the question of whether de facto compensation (25 Euros) would encourage blood donors to return to donate blood. The authors discovered that while compensated donors did return more frequently than uncompensated donors the difference between the two groups became insignificant in the third year after the initial donation. Note that since this survey focused on blood donation the reduction in return donors is likely to be lower than for plasma donation owing to the combination of a relatively similar degree of compensation for the two and the greater burden that the latter places upon donors.

64. Hartmann and Klein, "Supply and Demand for Plasma-Derive Medicinal Products – A Critical Reassessment Amid the COVID-19 Pandemic," 2750.

65. Nor would it reinforce their social degradation through the creation of a stigmatized class. As I will discuss in Chapter 6 there is no reason to believe that (at least within the United States) serving as a compensated plasma donor is stigmatized.

66. Other analyses of exploitation would also hold that some donors who donate plasma to plasma centers that operate in situations where they are prohibited from offering compensation would thereby be exploited by them. On Allen Wood's account of wrongful exploitation, for example, a person is exploited "when we treat their vulnerabilities as opportunities to advance our own interests or projects" and hence fail to provide them with the "[p]roper respect" that they are owed. (See Allen Wood, "Exploitation,"

Social Philosophy & Policy 12 (1995), 150. Legislators that prohibited donor compensation in the belief that some of the consequent shortfalls in the amount of plasma procured would be taken up by donors who would donate only when they believed that such a shortage would occur would exploit this class of donors in this way if it believed that they would advance their own interests through prohibition. Evidence that they – and the lobbyists that influence them – believe this is offered in Taylor, "The Ethics and Politics of Blood Plasma Donation."

6 Social Cohesion and Donor Approbation

Introduction

Ever since Richard Titmuss published *The Gift Relationship* it has been common for opponents of compensated donation rhetorically to ask whether a society in which persons are offered payment for their body parts is the sort of society in which we wish to live.[1] Since donor compensation is required to secure enough plasma to meet patients' medical needs, to enable certain donors to give their informed consent to their donation, to secure person's authoritative consent to the proposals that they are faced with, and to avoid exploiting the two classes of donors who are vulnerable to exploitation, the answer to this question should be a resounding "yes!". This is not the answer expected by those who ask this question. Instead, they expect "no" to be the answer. And often they expect this because they anticipate that those to whom this question is asked will believe that allowing donor compensation will somehow undermine social cohesion.[2]

The claim that allowing donor compensation will somehow undermine social cohesion is both widespread and frustratingly vague. The primary aim of both this chapter and the next is to rectify this. I will do so by taking up cudgels on behalf of those who *oppose* donor compensation by developing arguments for the view that allowing donor compensation would undermine social cohesion. Unfortunately for those who oppose donor compensation even the strongest arguments that are developed to support their view fail. There is thus no moral reason to oppose donor compensation – but plenty of moral reasons to support it.

Social Cohesion and the Avoidance of Hypocrisy

The development of persuasive arguments opposing donor compensation on the grounds that this would undermine social cohesion is not only important for the *moral* debate over donor compensation. It is also important for debate over public policy in countries that currently prohibit donor compensation (and not merely because moral arguments

DOI: 10.4324/9781003263913-7

should always be relevant for those who craft public policy). Many countries that prohibit donor compensation fail to procure a sufficient amount of plasma to produce the PDMPs that are required to meet the medical needs of their population. They thus import plasma (or PDMPs) to make up this shortfall – and do so from countries that allow donor compensation.

Consider, for example, the situation in Canada. Many provinces prohibit offering compensation to plasma donors but at the same time import plasma (and PDMPs) from the United States. They do this knowing that this was procured primarily from compensated donors. The situation in Quebec is illustrative.[3] This province has prohibited the financial compensation of donors since 1994.[4] As a consequence of this prohibition from 2013–2014 Quebec was only able to secure from domestic donors 14.5% of the intravenous polyvalent immunoglobulin (IVIg) that it needed.[5] To meet the medical needs of its population Quebec – a province ostensibly opposed to securing plasma from compensated donors – imported plasma from the United States knowing that some (if not all) of this was sourced from compensated donors. As Hema-Quebec noted in its Annual Report for that period "[t]he missing 85.5% of the volume . . . [was] . . . manufactured from plasma collected in the United States from paid donors (the law prohibits the compensation of donors in Québec)."[6] (Hema-Quebec is the organization that provides biological products of human origin – such as plasma – to hospitals in Quebec.) This was not an anomaly. In each year after 2013–2014, Quebec was unable to secure more than 21.5% of the immunoglobulin that it needed from uncompensated domestic donors. In each of these years the additional plasma that Quebec required "came from abroad, essentially the United States."[7] A similar story can be told for each of the other Canadian provinces that prohibit financially compensating plasma donors. For example, in the Parliamentary debate over Ontario's proposed ban on donor compensation it was acknowledged that approximately 70% of Ontario's immunoglobulin therapies are imported from the United States.[8] And at the national level Canadian Blood Services acknowledged (in 2020) that

> The amount of plasma we currently collect only meets about 13–14 per cent of the need for immune globulin (Ig), which is one of the plasma protein products in highest demand. The finished products we buy are made from plasma donated by paid donors in the United States.[9]

A similar story could be told for other countries that prohibit offering compensation to plasma donors but make up the consequent shortfalls in their supply by importing plasma from the United States. These include France,[10] Spain,[11] Sweden,[12] Portugal,[13] and the United Kingdom.[14]

It is telling that the value of United States exports of plasma products approaches $20 billion a year.[15]

Since these countries import plasma and PDMPs that they know are secured through donor compensation they cannot believe that plasma procured from compensated donors represents a health risk to patients. And since they are importing plasma from countries that allow donor compensation to make up the shortfall that results from their prohibition of this, they cannot believe that compensating donors will reduce the amount of plasma that is collected. Their objections to allowing donor compensation within their own borders must thus (as I noted in Chapter 1) be *ethical* objections. But to justify the prohibition of donor compensation *within* their borders while simultaneously accepting as legitimate the importation of plasma and PDMPs procured from compensated donors *outside* them requires that the ethical justification for the prohibition of domestic compensation must be of a particular type: One that can legitimate prohibiting compensation to persons within a certain geographical area but allowing compensation to take place outside it. Unless there is a morally relevant difference between persons within the borders of a country that prohibits donor compensation domestically but which considers it to be legitimate to import plasma secured from donors compensated outside them, then the same ethical considerations that would tell against compensating domestic donors would also tell against compensating foreign donors. The moral objection to compensating domestic donors thus cannot be based on (misplaced) concerns about informed consent, exploitation, or coercion. If offering compensation to donors undermines their ability to give their informed consent to donate, exploits them, or coerces them, then it will do so no matter which country they are in. A moral concern with social cohesion, however, *could* justify treating domestic donors differently from foreign donors. And it could do so without committing its proponents to the claim that social cohesion in *their* country (i.e., that which prohibits the compensation of domestic donors but allows the importation of plasma from compensated foreign donors) is more important than social cohesion in *other* countries (i.e., those that export their plasma).

The argument could progress as follows. (I am now paying off the promissory note that I issued in Chapter 1.) A high degree of social cohesion is valuable as this enhances the well-being of persons within the society that possesses it. The performance of actions that have a certain social meaning is necessary to cultivate and maintain social cohesion. In our society (i.e., that which prohibits the compensation of domestic donors but allows plasma to be imported from compensated foreign donors) the donation of plasma is an action that has the social meaning that is necessary to cultivate and maintain social cohesion.[16] We consider the donation of plasma to be the priceless gift of life. We also believe that for this reason plasma donors should never be compensated for their donations, for to do so would be to put a price on their priceless gift. Because plasma donors are never compensated in our society, the donation of plasma is understood by us to be an especially praiseworthy action selflessly performed for the good of others. Publicizing the existence of persons who donate their plasma without compensation encourages others to perform pro-social actions. We regard their pro-social actions to be heroic and encourage others to emulate them in any way they can. Encouraging pro-social actions cultivates and encourages social cohesion. But in our society charitable actions other than plasma donation are not as effective at encouraging others to behave in a prosocial manner as persons could be paid to perform them. (A soup kitchen worker could either be an unpaid volunteer, or someone who was paid for her work, for example.) Such actions thus have a different social meaning from those charitable actions for which, in our society, persons are never compensated (e.g., plasma donation). Introducing payment for goods or services that could previously only be secured through donation (e.g., plasma) would thus alter the meaning of the actions of their providers. If we allowed plasma donors to be compensated the provision of plasma would no longer be seen as a necessarily pro-social praiseworthy action. Its meaning would have changed. This would undermine the cohesiveness of our society by eliminating the most effective way we have of encouraging pro-social behavior. We should thus continue to prohibit compensating plasma donors. However, we recognize that this argument might only apply to our society. It is possible that the meanings of actions differ in other societies. It might be, for example, that a society that compensates its plasma donors places a different meaning on plasma donation than we do. They might see it merely as the provision of just another good while we see it as the giving of the priceless gift of life. (Perhaps they encourage social cohesion in other ways.) Thus, while we should continue to prohibit compensation for plasma donation to maintain social cohesion within *our* society given the meanings that we ascribe to certain actions we recognize that other societies might compensate their donors with no adverse effects on the cohesion of *their* societies. We thus prohibit the compensation of domestic donors while importing plasma and PDMPs from countries that maintain social cohesion in ways other than prohibiting donor compensation.

This is an elegant way to justify prohibiting compensating domestic donors while legitimizing the importation of plasma and PDMPs that are secured from donors compensated abroad. But four points should be noted before moving to develop and assess its claims concerning the relationship between social cohesion and donor compensation.

First, although the structure of this argument should make this clear it must be stressed that this argument is not intended to support the claim that a moral concern with social cohesion will *always* support the prohibition of compensated donation. Instead, it is intended only to support the claim that in *some* societies this concern will support this prohibition. This is not stacking the deck against those who oppose donor compensation *simpliciter*. The purpose of this argument was to justify the differential treatment of persons within a country's border (it is not permissible to encourage them to donate plasma through offers of compensation) and outside it (it is permissible to encourage them to donate plasma through offers of compensation). It is thus necessary for the purposes of this argument to admit the possibility that donor compensation is permissible even for persons concerned with promoting social cohesion.

Second, I have developed this argument for the benefit of those who oppose the compensation of domestic donors but who support the importation of plasma and PDMPs from countries that allow donor compensation. None of those who hold this position have offered this defense of it themselves. (Indeed, as far as I can tell no defense of this apparently hypocritical position has been offered at all.) It is thus part of my attempt to make the case against donor compensation as strong as possible – stronger even than the case that those who oppose donor compensation have made on their own behalf.

Third, while this argument could (if sound) theoretically justify the prohibition of donor compensation domestically while encouraging it abroad it is possible that the reasons that it gives for this differential treatment of domestic and foreign donors are *not* those that explain why these sets of donors are treated differently in practice. The actual reasons why a jurisdiction decides to prohibit allowing compensation to domestic donors while importing plasma and PDMPs that are known to be procured primarily from compensated donors abroad might have less to do with ethical concerns than with appeasing domestic interest groups that oppose donor compensation for their own interests. There is evidence that this is the case in Canada, for example. There, certain public service workers' unions oppose the compensation of domestic donors but do *not* similarly oppose the importation of plasma, or PDMPs, secured from donors they know were compensated as they fear that any increased commercialization of the domestic medical sector would threaten their economic self-interest.[17]

Finally, if it is admitted that there is nothing inherently wrong with offering compensation to prospective plasma donors, then any country that prohibits this would have to evaluate whether the costs of this are justified by the benefits. Thus, even if it is the case that the meaning of a plasma donation would change if compensated donation were to be introduced and this would, in turn, undermine social cohesion within the society in which this occurred, it is still an open question as to whether the benefits of compensated donation would outweigh the costs associated with this.[18]

Approbation or Compensation?

It is now time to develop arguments in favor of the view that a moral concern with social cohesion could justify the prohibition of donor compensation. I will develop the first of these arguments – the Argument from Approbation – in this chapter. I will then develop the second – the Contamination of Meaning argument that has been outlined by David Archard – in the next chapter.

Two Tenets of Market Faith

The earlier argument that I developed to support the view that the domestic prohibition of compensated donation could be justified within a jurisdiction that simultaneously encourages the compensation of foreign donors by allowing the importation of plasma (and PDMPs) known to be procured from compensated donors was based on the claim that the domestic prohibition of compensated donation was necessary to cultivate internal social cohesion. This was supported by the claim that a system of uncompensated plasma donation was necessary (in the society in question) to encourage the sort of pro-social actions that would contribute to social cohesion. Implicit in this argument was the denial of what Michael J. Sandel has termed "two tenets of market faith"[19] The first is that "commercializing an activity doesn't change it."[20] The second is that "ethical behavior is a commodity that needs to be economized."[21]

In response to the first of these tenets, Sandel noted that "commercializing blood changes the meaning of donating it."[22] He observes that if a donor were to be compensated $50 for a pint of blood a would-be altruist would be faced with questions that she would not be faced with were the donation of blood to be uncompensated. In a situation where persons were not financially compensated for donating blood this donor would be praised for donating a pint. However, if she donated a pint of blood without accepting financial compensation for this in a situation where a pint could secure the donor $50, then she might be *blamed* for donating. Her donation might be seen as selfish, securing her the warm glow of donation (and $50!) while precluding a needy person from securing $50 for donating blood. The offer of compensation has changed the meaning of her donation. The first tenet of market faith is thus false. Sandel also rejects the second tenet. Rather than seeing "[a]ltruism, generosity, solidarity, and civic spirit" as being like "commodities that are depleted with use" Sandel holds that they should be viewed "more like muscles that develop and grow stronger with exercise."[23] Although he provides no evidence for this claim it is certainly plausible. It is unlikely that each person has a certain reserve of these pro-social virtues that will be depleted with use. When combined with the rejection of the first tenet of market faith this view of the muscular nature of these pro-social virtues supports my earlier argument for the view that compensation should not be offered to the donors of blood or blood products.

Altruism and Approbation

The earlier argument for the view that a moral concern with social cohesion would (in a particular society) justify the prohibition of compensation for plasma donation agrees with Sandel that both of these tenets of market faith should be rejected. It first holds that introducing compensation for plasma donors into a situation where this had previously been prohibited would alter the meaning of subsequent plasma donation. (This claim will also form the basis of the Contamination of Meaning argument that I will discuss in the next chapter.) It combines this with the claim that the number of pro-social actions that are performed in a society could be increased or decreased depending on the beliefs and desires of the persons within that society.[24] With these claims in hand, it notes that a donor who donates plasma with no expectation that she will be compensated for this thereby indicates that she is concerned with the well-being of others. Others will approve of her for this. This approbation will encourage others also to act for the well-being of others, whether by donating plasma or in other ways. This, in turn, will enhance the cohesion of society by encouraging its members to care about each other's well-being. By contrast, a person who is compensated for her donation will not thereby indicate that she is concerned with the well-being of others. Her donation will thus not spur an increase in other-directed actions.[25] And if compensated donation is stigmatized in her society her donations might separate her from others. As a member of a stigmatized class, she will be considered by others to differ from them in an important way. She, in turn, will recognize her stigmatization and even if she rejects the value judgments that it is based on will view those who stigmatize her as being members of a class apart. Rather than merely failing to foster social cohesion allowing donor compensation could thus undermine it.

Furthermore, if a system of compensated donation was introduced into a society that had previously only allowed uncompensated donation the positive pro-social effects of uncompensated donation will be undermined by the presence of the former. (This approbation-based argument is of the type termed a "domino" argument by Margaret Jane Radin.)[26] The possibility of donor compensation would reduce the likelihood that any given donation would be taken to indicate that the donor was concerned with the well-being of others. Indeed, since it would likely be assumed that a person would prefer to receive compensation for her donation rather than not the default assumption would be that a donor had been compensated for her donation.[27] Uncompensated donors would thus be less likely to receive approbation from others for donating. Their donations would thus be less likely to spur others to perform similarly other-directed acts.

Moreover, if some uncompensated donors were motivated to donate (in whole or in part) by the degree of approval that they received from others the reduction in this that would likely result from the presence of a system of compensated donation would undermine their motivation to donate. A donor who would donate only if she received a certain degree of approbation would cease donating if the approbation that she received would be less than this after the introduction of a system of compensated donation. The introduction of a system of compensated donation into a society that had previously only allowed uncompensated donation could thus lead to a reduction in the number of persons who would be willing to donate without being compensated for doing so. This, in turn, would further undermine the likelihood that an uncompensated donor would receive the approval of third parties as it would lead to it being less likely that any given donor was uncompensated. This initial set of donors who ceased donating owing to the reduction in the level of approbation they received for this would thus be joined by another group of donors whose desired levels of approbation were now not being met. This further reduction in the number of uncompensated donors would further undermine the likelihood that uncompensated donors would receive approbation from third parties. The proportion of uncompensated donors in the donor population would thus continue to ratchet downward.

The focus of this argument is on the effects that the introduction of a system of compensated donation would have on the pro-social attitudes of the members of a society. It does not claim that the introduction of compensated donation would reduce the overall amount of plasma collected.[28] Its proponents could accept that the reduction in the amount of plasma procured from uncompensated donors could be offset by the correlative increase in the amount secured from compensated donors.[29] Nor does it make any claims about the relative numbers of opportunities that persons have for exhibiting pro-social behavior in systems where donation is uncompensated as compared to those where compensation is offered.[30] It is thus no response to it to note that the introduction of a system of compensated donation could increase the number of opportunities that persons would have to aid others – by, for example, accepting compensating for donating their plasma and then donating this to a charity.[31]

But while this argument is immune to these responses it still has serious deficiencies. Its soundness rests on the combined truth of several empirical claims: (1) That uncompensated donors who cease donating after the introduction of compensation will not substitute other pro-social activities in its stead; (2) that (financially) uncompensated donors will be primarily motivated to donate by the approbation they receive by doing so; (3) that the approbation accorded to uncompensated plasma donors will be significantly greater than that accorded to those who perform other pro-social activities without compensation; (4) that the approbation received by uncompensated donors will diminish once compensation is introduced; and (5) that compensated donors are stigmatized.³² But not only do these claims lack empirical support those that are crucial for the success of this argument are false.

Although the first of these claims is not explicit in the earlier argument it is necessary for it to be sound. If uncompensated donors cease donating after compensation is introduced but substitute in its place another pro-social activity for which they receive similar approbation their actions would continue to encourage others to behave in pro-social ways. They would thus continue to enhance social cohesion through encouraging pro-social behavior in others. Thus, for the introduction of donor compensation to undermine social cohesion by undermining uncompensated donation it must be the case that former donors who cease donating once compensation is introduced do not perform other pro-social activities in place of donation.

As I argued in Chapter 2 it is possible that some uncompensated donors will cease donating once compensation is offered as a result of coming to realize that their donations were not as valuable as they previously believed them to be. Such donors would be likely be motivated to find other ways find other ways (i.e., those whose value exceeded their opportunity costs of performing them) to express their pro-social motivations. This point can be generalized to other groups of uncompensated donors who cease donating once compensation is introduced. Those who were motivated to donate by the approbation that they received and who (for the reasons outlined earlier) would cease donating once compensation is introduced would also be likely to redirect their pro-social efforts so they continued to receive the approbation that they desired. Donors who (as discussed in Chapter 5) donated prior to the introduction of compensation as they believed that this was necessary to alleviate the shortage of plasma that they believed would result from the absence of compensation were donating to aid others. They, too, would thus be likely to redirect their pro-social actions into other avenues once compensation was introduced and, as a result, they came to believe that their donations were no longer necessary. If these claims concerning the redirection of (former) donors' pro-social activities are correct, then the first empirical claim that the soundness of the earlier argument depends upon will be false.

These claims are admittedly speculative. A defender of the earlier argument could readily challenge their veracity. But she would be ill-advised to do so. The approbation-based argument mentioned earlier is intended to support the view that the cohesiveness of a society would be enhanced were only uncompensated plasma donation to be allowed. To this end, it appealed to the view that persons who donated plasma without being compensated for so doing would thereby encourage both themselves and others to behave in other-directed, pro-social ways. The uncompensated donation of plasma was held to have a halo effect, motivating both plasma donors and those who were aware of their donations to behave more pro-socially in general. If this is true then if uncompensated plasma donors were to cease donating plasma once compensation was introduced, then it would be expected that they would redirect their pro-social efforts elsewhere rather than cease them altogether. As I discussed in Chapter 2 a person who donated plasma when no compensation for this was available might cease donating once compensation was introduced because this signaled to her that her donations were not as valuable as she had previously thought. Her cessation of donation once compensation is introduced thus should not be understood as signaling that she is now less pro-social than she was when compensation was prohibited. And, if the halo effect of uncompensated donation is true, it would be expected that such a donor would substitute other pro-social actions for plasma donation. If she did not do so – if she were *only* to express their pro-social motivations through uncompensated plasma donation – then the claim that the uncompensated donation of plasma contributed to social cohesion through motivating both donors and others to engage in other pro-social activities would be implausible.

The defender of the earlier argument against donor compensation within her society is thus caught on the horns of a dilemma. If she holds that the first empirical claim (1), mentioned earlier, is true, then her argument that prohibiting donor compensation is necessary to enhance social cohesion becomes implausible. But if she accepts that claim (1) is false (if she accepts that uncompensated donors could substitute other pro-social activities for plasma donation once compensation is introduced) then she has failed to provide a reason why the prohibition of donor compensation is necessary to encourage pro-social attitudes and social cohesion.

But the defender of the aforementioned argument might have a way to escape this dilemma. She could hold that persons who donate plasma when donor compensation is prohibited receive *far greater* approbation than persons who perform other pro-social actions. This is because, perhaps, the donation of plasma involves an invasive procedure whereas other pro-social activities (e.g., volunteering at a food bank) do not. Moreover, she could hold, the level of approbation accorded to uncompensated donors is needed to motivate others to perform other pro-social actions. They are, on this view, so impressed with the pro-social actions of uncompensated donors that while they do not believe that they can emulate them in performing the heroic act of plasma donation they do believe that they can emulate them in other, lesser, pro-social ways. With these claims concerning the distinct level of approbation accorded to uncompensated plasma donors in hand the defender of the argument could then claim that this level of approbation is necessary to motivate these donors to donate. Once donation is compensated, the level of approbation accorded to donors falls below the threshold necessary to motivate these approbation-hungry donors to donate. They thus not only cease donating but they also do not substitute any other pro-social actions for their donations. This decline in uncompensated donation serves to diminish other pro-social actions. Those who would perform these actions are no longer motivated to do so by a desire to emulate (to some degree) the acts of uncompensated donors.

This way of escaping the earlier dilemma relies on empirical claims (2), (3), and (4). But there is reason to believe that all of these claims are likely to be false. Claim (2) holds that uncompensated plasma donors would be primarily (if not exclusively) motivated to donate by receiving a high level of approbation. But the available empirical evidence does not bear this out. A study of donor motivation conducted in The Netherlands showed that persons who were considering becoming plasma donors were primarily motivated by a desire to engage in "helping others"; this was followed by a belief that they had a "responsibility to contribute to blood supply."[33] In descending order they were then motivated by "might need blood myself," "health check," "feeling proud," and "people dear to me needed blood."[34] The closest category in this study to the claim that uncompensated donors would be motivated to donate by approbation would be that of "feeling proud" (where this is understood as a form of *self*-approbation). This appears to have little effect on motivating persons to donate plasma when compared to other (pro-social) factors.[35] These results are concordant with those from a study of the motivations of whole blood and plasma and platelet donors in Quebec. The most common reason that plasma and platelet donors provided for donating was "My blood can save lives" (given by 77% of respondents), "Helping other people is in my nature" (given by 61% of respondents), and "It's a positive thing to do and requires little effort" (given by 52% of respondents).[36] Only 7% of respondents stated that they donated as "I feel recognition from people around me," although 45% did so as it made them feel proud.[37] Similar results have been found in an Australian study of whether whole blood donors would find converting to being plasma donors consistent with their identity as blood donors. It was discovered that many who decided to donate plasma "referred to helping others, feeling good about donating, and being a good citizen" as reasons for doing so.[38] A concern for others rather than a concern for one's own benefit ("[p]laisir, bien-être") was also reported by French plasma donors.[39]

This remarkable degree of cross-cultural consistency in the motivations of donors indicates that rather than being motivated to donate by a desire for approbation plasma donors are primarily motivated to donate by benevolence.[40] (This is concordant with their being motivated by the desire to "do the right thing" and receiving self-approbation as a result.) This directly undermines claim (2). And the truth of this claim was needed for the defender of the approbation-based argument mentioned earlier for the view that donor compensation must be prohibited to protect social cohesion to avoid the earlier dilemma. Moreover, this data also directly undermines claim (1): That if uncompensated donors ceased donating once compensation were introduced, then they would not substitute another pro-social benevolent action in its stead. (It also supports the claim made in Chapter 2: That the reason that donors cease donating once compensation is introduced is because they realize that their pro-social acts would have more value elsewhere.) And while this data does not undermine claim (3) (that the approbation accorded to uncompensated donors would be greater than that accorded to those who perform other pro-social acts without compensation) it does render it moot. This claim is only relevant if claims (1) and (2) should be accepted. And this data shows that they should not be.

Claim (4) (that the approbation received by uncompensated donors will diminish once compensation is introduced) is also rendered moot by this data. But this claim also faces further problems. On its face it is plausible. If some plasma donors are compensated a person will be less likely to praise someone that she learns is a donor than she would if no donors were compensated. She might assume that the donor was compensated for her donation and thus treat her as a vendor who had already secured her contracted due. But this scenario is based on two claims: That donors can be readily identified as such by third parties, and that there is no ready means of distinguishing compensated from uncompensated donors. Both of these claims are false. Unless one took it upon oneself to lurk outside plasma centers there would be no way for one to identify someone as a plasma donor unless she chose to identify herself as such. (She might, for example, wear clothing or jewelry that identifies her as a plasma donor – such as a T-shirt or a pin – or she might simply provide this information in conversation or on social media.) Donors who chose to identify themselves could then indicate whether they were compensated or uncompensated if this distinction was important to them. In a situation where compensated and uncompensated donation coexisted uncompensated donors who wished to identify themselves as such (perhaps because they believed that this would secure them approbation) could readily do so. And in such a situation it would not be implausible to hold that such donors would receive *more* approbation rather than *less* when compared to a situation where compensation was not allowed. They had, after all, not only donated their plasma – but to retain the purity of their gift had chosen to forgo the compensation that they were offered for this.[41]

The Myth of Stigmatized Compensated Donation

What, then, of the final empirical claim (5) implicit in the previous argument: That persons who accept compensation for their plasma donations are stigmatized? (Note that this claim is not necessary for the argument that uncompensated donation will *enhance* social cohesion; it merely functions to support the claim that compensated donation will *undermine* social cohesion.) This claim is repeated frequently in the literature on donor compensation. But despite its prevalence, there is remarkably little support given for it.

Most of those who claim that there is a stigma associated with compensated donation (of either blood or plasma) cite Richard Titmuss' *The Gift Relationship* and Martin J. Kretzmann's article "The Moral Stigmatization of Paid Plasma Donors" to support their view.[42] The first point to make here is that *The Gift Relationship* was published in 1970 and Kretzmann's article was published 1992. Moreover, both Titmuss and Kretzmann were writing of the (putative) stigma associated with receiving compensation for donation in the United States. And they were both writing of the stigmatization of compensated donors by medical professionals. Rather than supporting the claim that compensated donors are generally stigmatized Titmuss' and Kretzmann's work supports (at most) the claim that three decades ago compensated donors were stigmatized by (some) medical professionals in the United States. It does not support the claim that they are stigmatized now, or the claim that they are stigmatized outside the United States, or that they are stigmatized by persons other than medical professionals.

Second, and more importantly, neither Titmuss nor Kretzmann presents much evidence to support their claims that compensated donors are (or were) stigmatized. I will address Titmuss' claims first. Titmuss writes that "paid donors have been variously described . . . as narcotics, dope addicts, liars, degenerates, unemployed derelicts, prison narcotics users, bums, the faceless, the undernourished and unwashed, junkies, hustlers, and ooze-for-booze donors."[43] Titmuss cites a putative wealth of evidence in support of these stigmatizing descriptions, including papers in medical journals, conference proceedings, an article in a magazine aimed at medical professionals, and personal correspondence that he had received.[44]

But while this appears conclusively to establish that in the United States in the 1950s and 1960s medical professionals stigmatized compensated donors close examination of Titmuss' sources tells a different story.[45] Titmuss cites two personal communications, an article in the Weekly Report of the U.S. Department of Health, Education, and Welfare, an article from the *Wall Street Journal*, the magazine *Medical World News*, three articles from conference proceedings, and several articles in medical journals. The two personal communications are inaccessible – and in any case would provide evidence only of two person's prejudices against compensated donors rather than evidence of wider stigma associated with compensated donation. The Weekly Report that Titmuss cited makes no mention of compensated donation at all. Instead, it is merely a report of an outbreak of viral hepatitis among "known or suspected narcotics addicts" in a New Jersey county.[46] Similarly, the *Wall Street Journal* article that he cited noted only that a blood bank official objected to offers of compensation being made to plasma donors as he believed that this reduced the amount of whole blood that was donated to his bank.[47] It did not report that plasma donors were stigmatized in any way.[48]

The issue of *Medical World News* that Titmuss cited did refer to "Skid Row" donors.[49] But it does so in the context of a short humorous piece on how payment for plasma "is threatening to turn the Bowery Boys into the Bourgeoise" in the magazine's "Scissors and Scalpel" section of amusing anecdotes.[50] (Other pieces in this section included "No Fun in This Joint" on knee problems suffered by teenage girls as a result of dancing The Twist, and the lack of bananas at the National Institutes of Health as a result of a dock strike.)[51] The tone of the piece indicates that the author believes the offer of compensation to be a welcome opportunity for the "Bowery Boys" and that the term "Skid Row" was simply used as a colloquialism for the poor.

What of the three papers in conference proceedings that Titmuss cited? Although Titmuss appears to have cited the unpublished typescript versions of two of these works they can be readily identified. The first is Bernice M. Hemphill "The National Clearinghouse Program of the American Association of Blood Banks" in which she outlined how the program operated.[52] In this paper Hemphill mentions that "paid donors are more apt to provide false medical histories and identification than the voluntary donor who does not receive cash for his donation."[53] This does not establish that compensated donors were stigmatized. The second – from the same conference – is Charles B. Wheeler, Jr., "State Laws and Regulations."[54] Wheeler quotes from a paper published in the *New England Journal of Medicine*, August 13, 1964 that states that "alcoholic patients, drug addicts and other unreliable persons who deny disease for fear of rejection are attracted to any receptive and remunerative blood procurement center."[55] But prior to this quotation Wheeler explicitly noted that "there are good blood banks of each type [i.e., commercial and non-profit] and there are poor blood banks of each type."[56] He also noted that "some commercial banks are excellent institutions and that national blood needs require that such good commercial blood banks remain in operation."[57] Although Wheeler concludes that blood procured from commercial blood banks is "all things considered more dangerous than blood obtained from non-profit blood banks" his view is clearly not one that supports the stigmatization of compensated donors.[58] The third conference paper that Titmuss cites is "Malootian, I., *op. cit.*, 1964, p. 1002."[59] This cannot be found as cited. The only paper that Malootian published in 1964 made no mention of paid donors.[60] It seems that Titmuss was referring to Malootian's 1965 paper "A Plan to Attract Voluntary Blood Donors" which was first presented at a conference in Stockholm in 1964.[61] Malootian was critical of the increasing use of compensated blood donors in the United States on the grounds that they gave too frequently and "[t]hey are prepared spontaneously to answer 'no' to all of the medical history questions."[62] But she did not stigmatize them. Indeed, she *praised* them for refusing compensation for their blood once they were apprised of its value to the recipient.[63]

Of the papers in medical journals that Titmuss cited none disparage compensated donors in the way that he claims and only one (by R.F. Norris et al.) mentions (and that indirectly) the possible stigmatization of compensated donors. (This will be discussed later.) The earliest paper that Titmuss cited that discussed narcotic addition in the context of blood donation was a study of hepatic dysfunction and heroin addiction among incarcerated heroin addicts. The authors (Potter, Cohen, and Norris) noted that heroin addicts would pose a serious risk as blood donors owing to the increased incidence of hepatitis among them.[64] They also note that malnutrition could be a possible explanation for the abnormal liver functions of the incarcerated heroin addicts that they examined – although they noted that none had evidence of significant malnutrition.[65] They made no mention of compensated donation. A later paper cited by Titmuss (Adeshek and Adashek) that discussed compensated blood donation noted that in one study (by R.F. Norris) the incidence of hepatitis was similar to that discovered among narcotics addicts by Potter et al.[66] Adeshek and Adeshek also observed that other authors (P.I. Hoxworth et al., cited by Titmuss) had noted that hepatitis was more likely to be found among narcotics addicts and alcoholics than among the general population.[67] The conclusion drawn was that narcotics addicts who were willing to serve as donors for compensation would pose a risk to the blood supply. Adeshek and Adeshek also noted that such prospective donors would be motivated to dissemble about their medical history.[68] The other papers that Titmuss cite merely note the increased medical risks associated with securing blood (in the 1950s and 1960s) from compensated donors.[69] Titmuss' claim that the authors of the (accessible) works that he cited characterize compensated donors as "narcotics, dope addicts, liars . . . prison narcotics users . . . undernourished . . . junkies . . . and ooze-for-booze donors" is thus false.[70] Not only do many of the terms that he uses not appear in the (identifiable) works that he cited but those works are not providing evaluative accounts of the class of compensated donors as a whole. They either do not discuss compensated donors at all (e.g., Potter's work on imprisoned heroin addicts) or they are providing merely descriptive accounts of some subclasses of compensated donors.

The sole support that can be drawn from the work cited by Titmuss for the view that compensated donors were stigmatized in the 1960s is from R.F. Norris et al.'s discussion of the "Present Status of Hepatic Function Tests in the Detection of Carriers of Viral Hepatitis."[71] They observed that during their study at the William Pepper Laboratory of Clinical Medicine at the University of Pennsylvania the examining physicians "without conclusive proof" classified compensated blood donors "either as chronic alcoholics or narcotic addicts" when they returned for a follow-up visit.[72] At best, then, Titmuss' evidence establishes that in 1962 some physicians at the University of Pennsylvania Medical School harbored prejudices against a small subset of compensated donors.

Kretzmann's work similarly provides scant evidence for the claim that compensated donors are stigmatized. Kretzmann claims that his "[p]articipant observations in an urban plasma center" establish that "[p]aid plasma donors are subject to a distinctive moral stigma."[73] But his reported observations show no such thing. Kretzmann attended an urban plasma center in the Rocky Mountain area as a paid donor for eight weeks, spending five to eight hours a week in the setting.[74] He modelled his "appearance and behavior after the other young male donors" and at first interacted only with new donors; he then moved to talk with the "old hands."[75] He recorded how the staff at the center were suspicious of the paid donors – apparently suspecting them of substance abuse or of having medical problems that should preclude their donating – and stated that after his visit he felt "uncertain, angry, awkward, and anxious."[76] However, although Kretzmann repeatedly claimed that the "social meaning" of compensated plasma donation carried a "moral stigma," that "selling plasma is stigmatized because it is based on economic self-interest," that the staff considered the compensated donors to be "morally unworthy" and "second-class citizens," his reported observations do not bear this out.[77] Kretzmann reports that the staff of the center treated the donors as though they were concealing information and not to be trusted, and that some of the donors engaged in behavior that has been identified as that intended to counteract stigma.[78] However, he also noted that staff did not treat all donors in this way. College students were treated in a welcoming and friendly manner, as were regular donors.[79] The donors who were treated in the "stigmatized" were persons outside "respectable society" such as transients or the "mountain man" who made his living "trappin'" in the Rockies.[80] Rather than being stigmatized because they accepted compensation for their donations it appears that the typical donors in the center that Kretzmann attended were instead stigmatized for reasons independent of their receipt of compensation for their donations.

The approbation-based argument for the claim that fostering social cohesion through encouraging pro-social behavior would support the prohibition of donor compensation thus fails. None of the empirical claims that it is based on (1–5, mentioned earlier) are well founded. It is unlikely that uncompensated donors who cease donating after the introduction of compensation will fail to substitute other pro-social activities in its place. The available empirical evidence contradicts the claim that (financially) uncompensated donors will be primarily motivated to donate by the approbation that they receive as a result of doing so. Give the falsity of these two initial claims the truth of the claims that uncompensated donation will secure more approbation than other pro-social acts and that the approbation accorded such donors will diminish once compensation is introduced are moot. And there is no reason to believe that compensated donors are widely stigmatized *qua* compensated donors.

Conclusion

The claim that donor compensation should be prohibited to cultivate and maintain social cohesion is common in the literature on the ethics of compensating the donors of blood and blood products. But this claim is rarely supported by argument. This is unfortunate. Arguments against donor compensation that are grounded in the moral value of social cohesion could (if sound) legitimate the widespread practice of combining a prohibition on compensating domestic plasma donors with the active importation of plasma (and PDMPs) that is known to have been procured from compensated foreign donors. To aid those who endorse this asymmetric treatment of domestic and foreign donors I developed in this chapter an approbation-based argument for the view that a moral concern with the value of social cohesion could support the domestic prohibition of donor compensation. This argument failed. I will now turn in the next chapter to expand upon an alternative cohesion-based argument against donor compensation: The Contamination of Meaning argument that Archard developed from Titmuss' work.

Notes

1. See, for example, Keown, "The Gift of Blood in Europe," 97; Richard Fontaine, "Richard Titmuss on social cohesion: a comment," *European Journal of Political Economy* 20 (2004), 795–797. That Titmuss' work encouraged the view that "gifts" of blood and blood products would enhance social cohesion was recognized by Catherine Waldby and Robert Mitchell. *Tissue Economies: Blood, organs, and cell lines* (Durham, NC: Duke University Press, 2008), 19. However, they also recognized that "the form of the gift has no particular intrinsic powers of civil productivity, and offers no guarantees to . . . produce benevolent sociality" (ibid., 182).
2. See, for example, Campbell et al., "The Ethics of Blood Donation," 170. The claim that allowing donor compensation for blood would undermine social cohesion is also made by Angel Puyol, "Ética, Solidaridad y Donación de Sangre. Cuatro perspectivas para debatir," *Revista de Bioetica Derecho* 45 (2019), 51.
3. The following section of this paragraph is taken from Taylor, "The Ethics and Politics of Blood Plasma Donation," 92–93.
4. Bloodwatch, "Securing & Protecting The Canadian Blood Supply," 6.
5. Hema-Quebec, "Annual Report 2013–2014," 10. Available at: www.hema-quebec.qc.ca/userfiles/file/RA_2013-2014/HQ_RA_2013-2014_ANG_FINAL(1).pdf
6. Ibid.

7. Hema-Quebec, "Annual Report 2015–2016," 16. Available at: www.hema-quebec.qc.ca/userfiles/file/RA-2015-2016/RA_2015-2016_ANG-2.pdf. In 2014–2015 the figure was 83.9% ("from foreign sources"), in 2015–2016 80.3% of Quebec's immunoglobulin in 2016–2017 the figure was 79% ("with the rest coming from abroad"), and in 2017–2018 the figure was 78.5% "with the rest coming from the United States." See Hema-Quebec, "Annual Report 2014–2015," 15. Available at: www.hema-quebec.qc.ca/userfiles/file/media/anglais/publications/RA_2014-2015_ANG(2).pdf; Hema-Quebec, "Annual Report 2016–2017," 34. Available at: www.hema-quebec.qc.ca/userfiles/file/media/anglais/publications/AR_2016-2017_EN.pdf; Hema-Quebec, "Annual Report 2017–2018," 36. Available at: www.hema-quebec.qc.ca/userfiles/file/RA2017-2018/RA_2017-2018_EN_2.pdf.
8. Protein Plasma Therapeutics Association, "Updated Response to Ontario's Proposal to Ban Compensated Plasma Donation," Available at: www.pptaglobal.org/membership/current-members/28-news/ppta-news/900-ppta-s-updated-response-to-ontario-s-proposal-to-ban-compensated-plasma-donation.
9. Canadian Blood Services, "Our Commitment to Increasing Plasma Sufficiency in Canada," Available at: https://blood.ca/en/about-us/media/plasma/plasma-sufficiency
10. As Farrell observes while transfusionists in France claimed that they had achieved national self-sufficiency in blood and plasma products from VNRD by 1984 "(clandestine) importation of largely US-sourced plasma products in fact continued to meet the growing demand by PWH [people with hemophilia] throughout this period and beyond." Farrell, *The Politics of Blood*, 88.
11. Ll. Puig Rovira, "Plasma self-sufficiency in Spain," *Transfusion and Apheresis Science* 59, 1 (2020), 2. Available at: https://doi.org/10.1016/j.transci.2019.102700
12. Hannes Hansen-Magnusson, "Governance in the European Union: The European Blood Directive as an Evolving Practice," *Clinics in Laboratory Medicine* 30, 2 (2010), 493.
13. Laura Pricop, "Blood and Plasma Donors During the COVID-19 Pandemic: Arguments Against Financial Stimulation," *History and Philosophy of the Life Sciences* 43, Article 29 (2021), 2.
14. Ibid.
15. Sandro Ambuehl, Axel Ockenfels, and Alvin E. Roth, "Payment in Challenge Studies from an Economics Perspective," *BMJ Journal of Medical Ethics* 46, 12 (2020), 831.
16. The terms "our," "we," "theirs" and so on are simply used here for ease of exposition; they are not intended to refer to any particular polity.
17. See Taylor, "The Ethics and Politics of Blood Plasma Donation."
18. Owing both to the harms that the prohibition of donor compensation inflicts on patients and the wrongs that it inflicts both on donors and those who would operate plasma centers that would compensate their donors it is highly unlikely that the putative benefits of cultivating social cohesion by prohibiting donor compensation would outweigh its costs. For a similar point in the context of a discussion over organ markets, see Wilkinson, *Bodies for Sale*, 115.
19. Sandel, *What Money Can't Buy*, 125.
20. Ibid.
21. Ibid. 126.
22. Ibid. See, too, Archard's argument in the next chapter.

23. Ibid., 130. Peter Singer also famously denied that "ethical behavior is a commodity that needs to be economized," asking instead "Why should we not assume that altruism is more like sexual potency-much used, it constantly renews itself, but if rarely called upon, it will be begin to atrophy and will not be available when needed?" Peter Singer, "Altruism and Commerce: A Defense of Titmuss against Arrow," *Philosophy & Public Affairs* 2, 3 (1973), 319. Both Sandel and Singer are responding to Arrow's assertion that altruism is a scarce resource that should not be used up recklessly. Arrow, "Gifts and Exchanges," 355. For a discussion of the exchange between Titmuss, Arrow, and Singer see Taylor, *Stakes and Kidneys*, 167–173. Keown also endorses the view that altruism will expand with use rather than become depleted; see Keown, "The Gift of Blood in Europe," 97–98.

24. I use the term "pro-social" to avoid the problems associated with the "altruism" in the context of this debate – not the least of which are the worries that uncompensated donation is not necessarily altruistic, and that a focus on altruism illicitly assumes that all altruistic actions are thereby *prima facie* good. For a discussion of these issues see Hugh V. McLachlan, "The Unpaid Donation of Blood and Altruism: A Comment on Keown," *Journal of Medical Ethics* 24 (1998), 252–254.

25. John Keown offers an argument similar to this, although he does not draw out how prohibiting donor compensation will encourage pro-social actions through the approbation accorded to donors. John Keown, "A reply to McLachlan," *Journal of Medical Ethics* 24 (1998), 255–256.

26. Radin, *Contested Commodities*, 95.

27. This premise grants the existence of the first class of donors (discussed in the previous chapter) who are vulnerable to exploitation by plasma centers that are prohibited from offering compensation to their donors.

28. As noted by Julian Koplin, "From Blood Donation to Kidney Sales: The Gift Relationship and Transplant Commercialism," *Monash Bioethics Review* 33 (2015), 112.

29. See Chapter 1.

30. Koplin, "From blood donation to kidney sales," 112.

31. This response was made by Taylor, *Stakes and Kidneys*, 170, and Wilkinson, *Bodies for Sale*, 113–114.

32. The strength (but not the soundness) of this argument will also depend on what percentage of persons within the society in question would have their attitudes toward their fellows influenced by the means by which plasma was procured. If only a small percentage of the population would have their attitudes toward their fellows adversely affected by the introduction of donor compensation, then this argument would be weak, even if these empirical claims were correct.

33. Ingrid Veldhuizen and Anne van Dongen, "Motivational Differences Between Whole Blood and Plasma Donors Already Exist Before Their First Donation Experience," *Transfusion* 58, 3 (2012), 1682, Table 2.

34. Ibid.

35. Ibid.

36. Johanne Charbonneau, Marie-Soleil Cloutier, and Élianne Carrier, "Whole Blood and Apheresis Donors in Quebec, Canada: Demographic Differences and Motivations to Donate," *Transfusion and Apheresis Science* 53, 3 (2015), 324 Table 3.

37. Ibid.

38. Rachel Thorpe, Barbara M. Masser, Kyle Jensen, Nina Van Dyke, and Tanya E. Davison, "The Role of Identity in How Whole-Blood Donors Reflect on

and Construct Their Future as a Plasma Donor," *Journal of Community &
Applied Social Psychology* 30, 1 (2020), 78.

39. T. Schneider, O. Fontaine, and J.J. Huart, "Éthiques, motivations des donneurs d'aphérèse plasmatique," *Transfusion Clinique et Biologique* 11, 3
(2004), 149 Table 4.

40. For a discussion of the difference between benevolence and altruism in the
context of blood donation see E. Ferguson, K. Farrell, and C. Lawrence,
"Blood Donation is An Act of Benevolence Rather than Altruism," *Health
Psychology* 27, 3 (2008), 327–336.

41. This speculative claim – that donors who refused to receive financial compensation for donating when this was offered to them would believe that
this would secure them a greater of approbation if it were known that they
had donated without accepting financial compensation – is supported by
Mellström and Johannesson's observation that while the women in their
study were less likely to donate blood when offered financial compensation
to do so this effect was counteracted by the option of donating their payment
to charity. Mellström and Johannesson concluded from this that they were
motivated to donate by "social esteem" and this forgoing payment in this
way facilitated its receipt. Mellstrom and Johannesson, "Crowding Out in
Blood Donation," 847.

42. Titmuss, *The Gift Relationship*; Martin J. Kretzmann, "Bad Blood: The
Moral Stigmatization of Paid Plasma Donors," *Journal of Contemporary
Ethnography* 20, 4 (1992), 416–441. Titmuss' claims are cited by, for
example, Joel Schwartz, "Blood and Altruism," *Public Interest* 136 (1999),
41; Alexandra Kurlenkova, "Ova Exchange Practises at a Moscow Fertility
Clinic: Gift or Commodity?," in Olag Zvonareva, Evgeniya Popova, and
Klasien Horstman, eds., *Health, Technologies, and Politics in Post-Soviet
Settings* (London: Palgrave MacMillan, 2018), 175. Kretzmann's claims
are cited by, for example, Farrugia et al. "Payment, Compensation and
Replacement – The Ethics and Motivation of Blood and Plasma Donation,"
206 (Farrugia et al. do not endorse the claim that donors are stigmatized);
Kathleen Erwin, "The Circulatory System: Blood Procurement, AIDS, and
the Social Body in China," *Medical Anthropology Quarterly* 20, 2 (2006),
151; Kathleen Chell, Tanya E. Davison, Barbara Masser, and Kyle Jensen
"A Systematic Review of Incentives in Blood Donation," *Transfusion* 58
(2018), 252.

43. Titmuss, *The Gift Relationship*, 114–115.

44. Ibid., 114, note 5.

45. The suspect nature of Titmuss' scholarship here should raise questions about
the veracity of the rest of his work in *The Gift Relationship*. Outlining its
deficiencies is thus valuable. (See, too, the discussion in the previous chapter
of Titmuss' implausible account of how much blood donors were paid.)

46. W.J. Dougherty, "Narcotics Associated Hepatitis – New Jersey," *Morbidity and Mortality Weekly Report* 16, 21 (1967), 170. Titmuss miscites this
report.

47. Richard R. Leger, "Blood Shortage," *Wall Street Journal* (March 1, 1967).

48. Although it did report that when a blood bank attempted to incentivize
people to donate blood by offering baseball tickets "it was swamped by
both donors and protests. The protests came from persons who had donated
blood before the promotion and who didn't get tickets." Ibid.

49. Staff author, "Blood Money." Titmuss provided no bibliographic information about this article apart from the name and date of the magazine in
which it was published.

50. Ibid.
51. Staff author, "No Fun in This Joint," "Yes, We've Some Bananas," *Medical World News* (March 15, 1963), 136.
52. Bernice M. Hemphill, "The National Clearinghouse Program of the American Association of Blood Banks," *Proceedings of Conference on Blood and Blood Banking Drake Hotel, Chicago, December 11–12, 1964* (Chicago: Department of Environmental Health, American Medical Association, 1964), 75–81.
53. Ibid., 76. It is likely that Titmuss was working with an unpublished typescript of Hemphill's paper; this would explain the "p. 2" reference for this claim about "paid donors" on the second page of Hemphill's paper.
54. Charles B. Wheeler, Jr., "State Laws and Regulations," *Proceedings of Conference on Blood and Blood Banking Drake Hotel, Chicago, December 11–12, 1964* (Chicago: Department of Environmental Health, American Medical Association, 1964), 122–128.
55. Ibid., 125. Although Wheeler does not cite his source, he is quoting George F. Grady, Thomas C. Chalmers, and The Boston Inter-Hospital Liver Group, "Risk of Post-Transfusion Viral hepatitis," *New England Journal of Medicine* 271, 7 (1964), 341.
56. Wheeler, "State Laws and Regulations," 125.
57. Ibid.
58. Ibid.
59. Titmuss, *The Gift Relationship*, 114, note 5.
60. Ida Malootian, "The 'Emergency' Requisition," in L.P. Holländer, ed., *International Society of Blood Transfusion. 9th Congress, Mexico, September 1962: Proceedings* (Basel: Karger, 1964, vol. 19), 696–699.
61. Ida Malootian, "A Plan to Attract Voluntary Blood Donors," in L.P. Holländer, ed., *International Society of Blood Transfusion. 10th Congress, Stockholm, September 1964: Proceedings Part IV: Advances in Blood Transfusion / Treatment of Erythroblastosis Foetalis / Automation / New Equipment / Hepatitis Problems* (Basel: Karger, 1965, vol. 23), 1002–1005.
62. Ibid., 1002.
63. Ibid., 1003.
64. H. Phelps Potter, Jr., Norman N. Cohen, and Robert F. Norris, "Chronic Hepatic Dysfunction in Heroin Addicts: Possible Relation to Carrier State of Viral Hepatitis," *Journal of the American Medical Association* 174, 16 (1960), 2049–2051.
65. Ibid., 2050.
66. Eugene P. Adashek and William H. Adashek, "Blood-Transfusion Hepatitis in Open-Heart Surgery," *Archives of Surgery* 87, 5 (1963), 794. Adashek and Adashek cite R.F. Norris, "Present Status of Hepatic Function Tests in the Detection of Carriers of Viral Hepatitis," *Paper Presented at IXth International Congress of Society of Blood Transfusion, Mexico City* (September 1962), and "The Carrier of Viral Hepatitis as a Blood Donor," in *Proceedings of the VIIIth Congress of the International Society of Blood Transfusion, 1960* (White Plains, NY: Albert J. Phiebig Books, 1962), 37–44.
67. Adashek and Adashek, "Blood-Transfusion Hepatitis in Open-Heart Surgery," 794, P.I. Hoxworth et al. "The Risk of Hepatitis From Whole Blood and Stored Plasma," *Surgery, Gynecology, & Obstetrics* 109 (1959), 38–42.
68. Adashek and Adashek, "Blood-Transfusion Hepatitis in Open-Heart Surgery," 794
69. Titmuss, *The Gift Relationship*, 114, note 5.
70. Ibid., 114–115.

71. Norris et al., "Present Status of Hepatic Function Tests in the Detection of Carriers of Viral Hepatitis," 202–210.
72. Ibid., 207.
73. Kretzmann, "Bad Blood," 416.
74. Ibid., 420.
75. Ibid.
76. Ibid., 424–425, 426.
77. Ibid., 416–417; the phrase "second class citizens" occurred on 432.
78. Ibid., 423, 429–430.
79. Ibid., 433–434, 429.
80. Ibid., 429.

7   Contamination, Cohesion, and Imagined Community

Introduction

In the previous chapter, I developed an argument in favor of prohibiting donor compensation that was based on the value that this would putatively have for maintaining social cohesion. This argument was based on the claim that allowing donor compensation would (in some societies) reduce some person's motivation to donate plasma, with this, in turn, more generally undermining persons' motivations to behave in pro-social ways. The prohibition of donor compensation was thus held to cultivate and encourage social cohesion through cultivating and encouraging pro-social behavior. I argued that this approbation-based argument failed.

But that argument is not the only argument from the "social meaning" of donation that could be marshalled against allowing donor compensation. In this chapter, I will consider another such argument – the Contamination of Meaning argument that David Archard developed from Titmuss' work in *The Gift Relationship*. After outlining Archard's account of the Contamination of Meaning argument I will develop it further to ensure that I address the strongest version of this argument that could be offered to support the views of those who believe that a moral concern with social cohesion will support the prohibition of donor compensation. In so doing I will explain why the prohibition of compensation for the donation of blood and blood products could be especially important for social cohesion. But even this developed version of the Contamination of Meaning argument fails. Its justification for giving special treatment to blood and blood products turns out to be self-defeating. And the available empirical evidence casts further doubt on the claim that allowing donor compensation undermines social cohesion.

The Tottering Domino of Social Cohesion

The Contamination of Meaning argument begins with the premise that "With respect to some good, P, one must think of P in either exclusively monetary terms (P is priced) or exclusively nonmonetary terms

DOI: 10.4324/9781003263913-8

(*P* is priceless, without price, beyond price)."[1] The second premise is that "the effect of a market in *P* . . . is that *P* comes to be thought of in dominantly if not exclusively monetary terms."[2] Thus, the proponents of this argument conclude, "the market in *P* comes to dominate in the sense that there is no opportunity for a pure 'gift' of *P*, the donation of *P* being equivalent to the transfer of its monetary value."[3] Archard explains that on this view the monetary value associated with the sale of blood will also become associated with blood that is donated changing the meaning of the donation from one that was previously "priceless" to one that was the equivalent of a monetary donation. The meaning of donations would thus become "contaminated" by the presence of the market.[4]

Archard notes that the conclusion of this argument is not that persons would be less motivated to give blood as a result of the contamination of such gifts' meanings by the presence of donor compensation.[5] Rather, its conclusion is that the meaning of the fee-free donations given in the presence of donor compensation would be altered for the persons who recognized the possibility of compensation. Such donations would no longer be gifts without price but would be gifts that had a particular price. A donation of blood or plasma would be the equivalent of a monetary donation of a set amount.

This matters for social cohesion in the following way. Being a member of a community is "a way of being with others."[6] Other relationships will provide other ways of being with others. Familial relationships and relationships between friends are all ways of being with others – as are the relationships that hold between the participants in a market. The norms that structure these relationships differ. It would, for example, be inappropriate within contemporary American society for friends to keep track of favors that they had done for each other with the expectation that the score would be made even. But this form of interpersonal accounting could be highly appropriate for persons in a small farming community. Such favor-trading could foster both fellow-feeling as well as diminish the likelihood of long-term resentments that could be engendered by one person taking advantage of another. Consider, for example, James Rebanks' account of business transactions in the sheep-farming communities of England's Lake District.[7] When one member of the community made a deal with another that turned out to be especially advantageous for her, she was expected to trade with him again in the future in such a way that he would be benefitted to the same degree. By contrast, in a purely business relationship (even one between persons who expected to repeat their interactions) such a windfall benefit would not engender any obligation for repayment on the part of she who received it.

Some of the norms that govern how persons are to be with others thus govern whether and in what way they should consider the costs and benefits that they incur and receive in their relationships. Certain types of relationships are so constituted that those involved in them naturally relate to each other without any consideration of the costs and benefits of so doing. The loving spouses of O'Henry's story "The Gift of the Magi" were in a relationship of this sort; they "sacrificed for each other the greatest treasures of their house."[8] Their love led them to be concerned only with the other's interests and so silenced considerations of any costs they would incur in so doing. In other relationships – such as those that are "all business" – concern about costs and benefits are (appropriately) paramount. The role that considerations of costs and benefits play in these two types of relationships are both clearly defined and readily adhered to. Yet other types of relationships are more liminal and the degree to which costs and benefits feature (or should feature) in them is more susceptible to revision. Such relationships would need to be actively sustained as a particular type of relationship to prevent them from changing into one that was different. The relationships that exist between the sheep farmers of the Lake District might be of this sort. Some persons in this community might decide to treat farming more as a business than as a way of life. For them, windfall profits would not need to be repaid in the future to those from whom they were secured. Over time, these norms might crowd out the more community-orientated norms that had preceded them. (The more business-orientated farmers might be more commercially successful and so acquire the means to buy out their more traditional neighbors, or the more traditional farmers might decide to adopt the norms of their business-orientated neighbors to protect themselves from being taken advantage of.) In such a way a close-knit community of persons engaged in a shared agricultural way of life could transform into a community of individual businesses. To guard against this possibility the members of the community might need to impose informal sanctions (e.g., by refusing to deal with them, either socially or professionally) on those who attempted in this way to change the norms that governed how costs and benefits featured in their individual deliberations.

The need to police certain types of relationships to ensure that those party to them do not change their view of the appropriate role that considerations of costs and benefits play in them is the key to understanding how the Contamination of Meaning version of the domino argument against donor compensation is intended to work. The relationships between the spouses in "The Gift of the Magi" and the traders who considered themselves to be related "only for business" needed no policing to continue as they were. The appropriate role that considerations of costs and benefits played in them was transparent to their participants (i.e., irrelevant to the former, the focus of the latter) and owing to their immersion in their relationships the question of whether they should alter this would not arise. But other relationships (such as, perhaps, that of the Lake District sheep farmers) will require policing to guard against transformation. Relationship policing would be relatively unchallenging in a situation where those party to the relationship would both be in proximity to each other and would frequently interact (as is the case of the sheep farmers). It would be more challenging – and hence the desired relationship between those party to it more difficult to sustain – if these conditions did not hold.

This is the case with what Archard identified as an "imagined community" whose members are spread across a significant geographic area and where the particular relationship that holds between them that constitutes it is sustained by their belief in its nature.[9] Unlike the loving spouses of "The Gift of the Magi" the members of an imagined community (such as a nation) would not automatically be immersed in a particular relationship to each other.[10] They might see themselves as individuals associated by mere geographical happenstance. If this is the case, then they might believe that their relationship is and should be one where each looks after his own interests with considerations of costs and benefits playing a central role in their interactions. Alternatively, they might see themselves as constituting a community (e.g., "the Scots") having certain shared ends which transcend considerations of the costs and benefits that might be incurred or received by them as individuals. The different ways of understanding the type of community that they belong to would be reflected in how the persons concerned interact with each other. Since some forms of interaction would (overall) be more beneficial to them than others it would be preferable for them to adopt an understanding of their community that would facilitate these. If such a beneficial understanding would be cultivated by limiting the degree to which they assess their individual actions in terms of the costs and benefits that they incur and receive as individuals instead of focusing on the ways in which their actions would contribute to the community as a whole this would give them reason to foster it by imposing this limitation.

One way to foster a relationship in which considerations of costs and benefits play a background role (or no role at all) in a situation where those party to the relationship would not automatically ignore them (or pay little attention to them) is to make it more difficult for these considerations to apply. Precluding the pricing of the goods that would be exchanged within this relationship would assist here. To motivate the members of a polity to interact with others *qua* members of that polity, and hence to see their interactions as being unmediated by considerations of individual costs and benefits, the goods that they would exchange *qua* members of that polity should be unpriced. Markets in political goods exchanged between the members of this polity *qua* members of this polity (such as votes or access to members of Congress) should thus be prohibited.[11] For the same reason markets in other goods that could in principle be both provided by all and needed by all (e.g., blood or plasma) could also be prohibited. This would encourage their exchange among the members of the polity (and, in principle, between *all* the members of the polity with no one group in principle being givers and one being the recipients) without invoking considerations of costs incurred and benefits received. While allowing such goods to be priced would not preclude the possibility of their donation it could change the meaning of the good donated from being one that is priceless to being one that is priced. If this occurred this change in meaning would both facilitate and invite the members of the polity to judge the costs and benefits that accrue to them as individuals from the exchange of these goods. This, in turn, would encourage them to see their relationship with other members of the polity in terms where considerations of costs and benefits to them as individuals were foregrounded rather than quieted. Allowing or precluding the pricing of certain goods could thus partially determine the type of relationship that members of a polity consider themselves to be party to *qua* members of that polity. If a more morally desirable relationship between them could be fostered by preventing the overt pricing of certain goods, then this would provide a reason to prevent the pricing of those goods. Hence, if blood or plasma are goods whose pricing should be prevented to foster this type of political relationship then (assuming that the value of this end would warrant this, when compared to the costs that it might impose upon the members of the polity) donor compensation should not be allowed.

The Gift of Blood and the Imagined Community

I have drawn on Archard's construal of Titmuss' argument to develop the aforementioned argument. As before in this volume, I have done this to address the most developed and persuasive version of a common claim offered by those who oppose donor compensation. But even though this is the most developed and persuasive version of the "Contamination of Meaning" argument we should still refrain from accepting it.[12] Archard recognized that considerable work needs to be done to elaborate his form of this argument before it should be accepted.[13] This hesitancy also applies to the more developed form of this argument that appears earlier. In the argument outlined earlier it was held that the prohibition of donor compensation was necessary to contribute to the preservation of the type of relationship between the members of a polity that it would be desirable for them to have. To be persuasive this argument would need to provide both a detailed descriptive account of this relationship as well as a normative defense of its desirability. It would also need to provide an account of why the prohibition of compensation for the donation of blood and blood products is necessary for the society at issue to contribute to the preservation of this type of relationship between its members. This descriptive account of the political relationship would emphasize social solidarity. The members of the polity would identify with their membership of it and as a result have a sense of belonging. They would consider themselves to owe loyalty to their fellow members, and hence have obligations to support them. They would trust their fellow members and would consider them to be their moral equals in all important moral and political respects.[14] Having this type of relationship with their fellows would be of value to the members of the polity. The sense of belonging that it would provide to them would contribute to their sense of security and their well-being.[15] Their well-being and sense of security would also be enhanced by their ability to trust their fellow members and their justified expectation that they would provide them with aid as needed. Their shared view of their moral and political equality would minimize conflict within the polity and contribute to their sense of self-worth.

Problems With This View

Yet while it is relatively straightforward to offer an overview of the type of relationship that it would be beneficial for the members of a polity to have with each other defending the view that its maintenance in any given society would require a prohibition on donor compensation is far more challenging. Some indication of how such a defense might proceed was indicated earlier and will be elaborated here. The members' expectation that others would aid them in time of need could require that they be relatively insensitive to considerations of the costs that they would incur and benefits that they would receive from aiding each other. To support the view that some of their interactions should not be determined by considerations of costs and benefits a space should be made for them to exchange unpriced goods. To cultivate the expectation that they would receive aid from their fellow members in times of need institutions should be in place to both facilitate and publicize such aid. To support further the view that the members of the polity are equal in morally important respects these institutions should focus upon facilitating securing and distributing aid that all members of the polity could in principle provide, and that all might in principle require. This approach would emphasize their equality by eliminating the possibility of their division into a class of persons who provided aid and a class who received it. These ends could all be achieved through prohibiting compensation being offered to, for example, the donors of blood or plasma. A blanket prohibition on compensating the donors of blood or plasma would effectively secure a space for the provision of unpriced goods that could be insulated from any possible price contamination from a shadow market. Moreover, these are goods that, in principle, all could contribute, and that, in principle, all might need. The concern to cultivate and preserve the type of desirable political relationship that was outlined earlier between the members of a polity could thus justify the prohibition of donor compensation.

But while this tentative account of how such a defense of the prohibition of donor compensation would develop provides it with some initial plausibility it also faces serious problems. While blood and plasma might appear to be especially well suited to emphasize the equality of the members of the polity prohibiting their donors from receiving compensation comes at a considerable cost: It results in far less plasma being collected than would have been had procured had compensation been allowed.[16] This, in turn, places a significant burden on those members of the polity who are dependent on plasma and PDMPs. Thus, while the prohibition of donor compensation might appear to emphasize the equality of the members of the polity it does not actually do so for it imposes significant costs on a particular identifiable subset of them. As an approach to communicate the equality of the members of the polity this is directly self-defeating.

It also seems doubtful that the desirable features of the relationship outlined earlier would be associated in any way with a prohibition of donor compensation.[17] If it were true that prohibitions on donor compensation within a polity would encourage cohesion between its members that would encourage trust and mutual aid, then we would expect polities that allowed donor compensation to exhibit *lower* degrees of social trust and charitable giving than those that prohibited this. But this is not the case. Although the United States allows plasma donors to be compensated it is ranked as a medium-trust society, with 36% of its population trusting other people.[18] (It places 16th out of 60 nations surveyed.)[19] More strikingly, the United States has consistently ranked for a decade as the country with the most generous citizens, with 58% saying that they had helped a stranger, donated money, or volunteered time.[20] By contrast, while France prohibits the compensation of plasma donors it ranks as a low-trust country, with only 23% of its population trusting other people.[21] It also ranks 66th out of 125 countries with respect to the generosity of its citizens.[22] Lest one think that there is a correlation between social trust, generosity, and compensated donation, Canada (where donor compensation is widely prohibited) is a high-trust country (placing joint 4th out of 60 nations surveyed) with a high degree of generosity among its citizens (placing 5th out of 125 countries).[23] This lack of correlation between the allowance or prohibition of donor compensation, social trust, and generosity casts doubt on any claim that prohibiting donor compensation would have a significant causal effect on the relationship that the members of the polity concerned have with each other.

A Better Alternative

Recognition of the difficulties associated with the aforementioned approach to cultivating and sustaining a particular view of the relationship that should be shared by the members of the imagined community of the polity raises the question of whether an alternative approach would be better.

The earlier discussion focused on the question of how to cultivate a relationship between the members of the imagined community of a polity understood as a political organization governed by a particular set of laws (e.g., those that prohibited donor compensation). This focus was a natural result of addressing the question of whether compensation for blood and plasma should be prohibited. This way of framing the issue naturally directs the discussion of it into a discussion of whether a polity with a particular legal system should allow donor compensation. But questions that concern which relationships the members of an imagined community should have with one another can focus on communities that extend beyond the boundaries of the nation-state. (One might, for example, be concerned with the imagined community of all persons who donate plasma and the patients who benefit from this.) And there is *prima facie* reason to believe that focusing on an extra-national imagined community would be morally preferable to focusing on a community identified with a nation-state. The political boundaries of a nation-state have no moral significance. Emphasizing them as the locators of a moral community would thus, without further argument, be unjustified. An imagined community that is identified by the characteristics of its members rather than the artificial bounds of a polity would accordingly be more morally justifiable. Rather than aiming to cultivate social cohesion among the members of a polity, it would thus be morally preferable to cultivate it between the members of a nonpolitical imagined community. Pursuing cohesion among the members of such an imagined community could not be readily achieved through legal means for its membership would straddle different legal jurisdictions. The cultivation and preservation of an appropriate relationship between the members of this community would thus need to be advanced through other means. Consider, for example, the cultivation of an imagined community that consists of persons who have benefitted each other through trade. This community would consist of some persons who have traded face to face (e.g., a shopper and the owner of a local grocery store). But it would also consist of persons who have never met each other (e.g., the packer of a consumer's Amazon order and its recipient, or a child in the United States and a worker in the Chinese factory that made her sneakers).

This imagined community would be both global and exceptionally diverse. It could be developed by persons coming to realize just how many others contributed to the production and distribution of the goods that they enjoy, whether they enjoy these as a member of the affluent West or as a consumer in a relatively impoverished area of the global South. Education would need to play a central role in demonstrating the global supply chains that link the people of this global community together in webs of mutual dependence and benefit.[24] Education would also be needed to demonstrate that market transactions are (at least *ex ante*) positive rather than zero sum games. And it would be needed to show that just as blood and plasma could, in principle, be provided by anyone and needed by anyone, so too does the fact of comparative advantage provide everyone with the opportunity to contribute to increasing the well-being of the trading community. Rather than the offer of compensation undermining social cohesion it could instead be used to cultivate and sustain it across the imagined community of the beneficiaries of trade. In this community, a concern with costs and benefits would not rend asunder the ties that bind its members together as parties to a desirable relationship. Instead, though emphasizing their role in signaling to its members through prices where they should direct their efforts for the good of themselves and others, considerations of costs and benefits could draw persons closer together in their shared pursuit of well-being.

Conclusion

In the last chapter, I attempted to support the view of those who hold that offering compensation for the donation of plasma would undermine social cohesion. The argument that I outlined there held that reducing the approbation that persons within this society would receive for their pro-social actions would undermine their motivation to perform them. But, despite my best efforts, this argument failed. Undeterred, in this chapter, I developed an alternative domino argument against donor compensation that was also grounded on a moral concern for the value of social cohesion. This, too, has failed. While these failures do not show that a moral concern for social cohesion cannot justify the prohibition of donor compensation, they do show that we should, at least, be skeptical of such claims. This skepticism is important. I argued in the previous chapter arguments against donor compensation that are grounded on a moral concern with social cohesion would be those that should be drawn upon to justify an asymmetric policy whereby compensation should be prohibited domestically but plasma (and PDMPs) from donors known to be compensated for their donations could be imported. The failure of these cohesion-based arguments should lead to a revision of this policy. And since (as I have argued in this volume) allowing donor compensation is morally required there is no reason for any country with a suitable donor population to continue to prohibit this.

Notes

1. David Archard, "Selling Yourself: Titmuss's Argument against a Market in Blood," *Journal of Ethics* 6, 1 (2002), 93. This account of Archard's view is taken from James Stacey Taylor, *Markets with Limits: How the Commodification of academia derails debate* (New York: Routledge, forthcoming), Chapter 5.
2. Archard, "Selling Yourself," 94.
3. Ibid.

4. Ibid., 95. Emphasis added.
5. Ibid. See my similar comment about the approbation-based argument I developed in the previous chapter.
6. Ibid., 97. What follows is a version of a Contamination of Meaning argument that has been suggested by Archard's work, but which is not intended to be a reconstruction of an argument that he developed.
7. James Rebanks, *The Shepherd's Life: A Tale of the Lake District* (London: Allen Lane, 2015), 23–25.
8. O. Henry, "The Gift of the Magi," in O. Henry, ed., *O'Henry Stories* (New York: Platt & Munk, 1962), 48.
9. Archard, "Selling Yourself," 92. Archard cites Benedict Anderson, *Imagined Communities: Reflections on the Origin and Spread of Nationalism* (London: Verso, 1983), 14–16.
10. See Archard's discussion in "Selling Yourself," 100–102.
11. See Sandel, *What Money Can't Buy*, 22–23.
12. Jason Brennan and Peter Jaworski have argued against Archard's "Contamination of Meaning" argument on the grounds that it is a "semiotic" objection–one that holds that independently of concerns about exploitation, misallocation, rights, paternalism, harm to others, or corruption,

> to allow a market in some good or service X is a form of communication that expresses the wrong attitude toward X or expresses an attitude that is incompatible with the intrinsic dignity of X, or would show disrespect or irreverence for some practice, custom, belief, or relationship with which X is associated.
>
> (Jason Brennan and Peter M. Jaworski, *Markets Without Limits: Moral Virtues and Commercial Interests* (New York: Routledge, 2016), 47)

> Brennan and Jaworski correctly argue that all semiotic objections to markets (and hence to the exchange of money for goods and services) fail (ibid., Part II). But this objection does not touch Archard's Contamination of Meaning argument for this is not a semiotic objection to compensation as Brennan and Jaworski define these. See Taylor, *Markets with Limits*, Chapter 5.

13. Archard, "Selling Yourself," 102–103.
14. I follow Julian J. Koplin in adopting Meena Krishnamurthy's account of political solidarity from Krishnamurthy's, "Political Solidarity, Justice and Public Health," *Public Health Ethics* 6(2), 129–141. See Koplin, "From Blood Donation to Kidney Sales," 108.
15. See, for example, Michael Skey, "Why do Nations Matter? The Struggle for Belonging and Security in an Uncertain World," *The British Journal of Sociology* 64, 1 (2013), 81–98.
16. See the discussion in Chapter 1. The claim that blood and plasma are well-suited to emphasize equality in this way is not an essentialist semiotic claim but one indexed to the likely meanings associated with these goods in the contemporary United States.
17. Alastair V. Campbell expresses similar skepticism about the efficacy of prohibiting donor compensation to facilitate social cohesion. After noting that "solidarity" is a "key socio-political concept" in "many European countries" he notes that while "these countries also have a prohibition on the sale of blood and other body parts . . . this hardly proves a causal relationship between the two!" Alastair V. Campbell, *The Body in Bioethics* (New York: Routledge-Cavendish, 2009), 21. Campbell goes on to note that "the

presence or absence of a voluntary blood donation system surely could not have the normative effect suggested by Titmuss" (ibid.).

18. Jan Delhey and Kenneth Newton, "Predicting Cross-National Levels of Social Trust: Global Pattern or Nordic Exceptionalism?" *European Sociological Review* 21, 4 (2005), 315.

19. Ibid.

20. Charities Aid Foundation, *CAF World Giving Index 2019* (West Malling, Kent: Charities Aid Foundation, 2019), 7.

21. Delhey and Newton, "Predicting Cross-National Levels of Social Trust," 315.

22. Charities Aid Foundation, *CAF World Giving Index 2019*, 24.

23. Delhey and Newton, "Predicting Cross-National Levels of Social Trust," 135; Charities Aid Foundation, *CAF World Giving Index* 2019, 23.

24. For an excellent example of this see Leonard E. Read, *I, Pencil* (Atlanta, GA: Foundation for Economic Education, 2019).

Conclusion

The debate over the morality of offering financial compensation to persons in an attempt to increase the medical supply of human bodily parts and services has worked its way into a familiar groove. The opponents of donor compensation offer a series of reasons as to why the procurement of bodily materials and services from uncompensated donors would be instrumentally superior to procuring them from compensated donors, or else (where this is an inclusive or) they argue that this practice is sufficiently immoral to justify its prohibition. In response, the defenders of donor compensation argue that the procurement of bodily parts and services from compensated donors leads to better results than allowing only their procurement from uncompensated donors, or (again, an inclusive or) that the ethical objections leveled against this practice are misplaced. On encountering a new contribution to this debate one might well wearily recall Ecclesiastes 1.9 – "What has been will be again, what has been done will be done again; there is nothing new under the sun."[1]

This volume changes that. It does not merely defend the view that it is ethically acceptable to offer compensation to plasma donors. It goes on the offensive, arguing that it is the *prohibition* of donor compensation that is unethical. As I argued in Chapter 1, the most important point to note here is that the prohibition of donor compensation harms patients by reducing their access to safe PDMPs. I also argued that the legal prohibition of donor compensation wrongs donors. As I argued in Chapter 2 prohibiting donor compensation undermines the ability of some donors to give their informed consent to donate. In addition to this, proposals to prohibit donor compensation would, as I argued in Chapter 3, fail to secure the authoritative consent of either prospective donors or the prospective operators of commercial plasma centers. Subjecting these persons to them would thus wrong them. By contrast, allowing donor compensation would respect the authoritative consent of all parties to the proposals involved in it and so would not be wrongful. And (as I argued in Chapter 5, drawing on the account of exploitation that I developed in Chapter 4) while the prohibition of donor compensation would lead to

DOI: 10.4324/9781003263913-9

the exploitation of some donors allowing donor compensation (as this is currently practiced in the United States and Europe) would not.

The instrumental and ethical concerns that are often offered as reasons to prohibit donor compensation thus not only fail to justify the prohibition of donor compensation: When taken seriously they establish that it is the *prohibition* of donor compensation that is unethical. These instrumental and ethical concerns also fail to justify the approach to plasma procurement that has been adopted in many countries: The practice of prohibiting domestic plasma centers from offering donor compensation while allowing the importation of plasma (and PDMPs) from foreign donors that are known to have been compensated. If it is (falsely) believed that offering compensation to donors would be sufficiently wrongful to justify its legal prohibition, or (again, falsely) that plasma (or PDMPs) from compensated donors imposes health risks on patients, then it seems that steps should be taken to prevent or discourage donor compensation (e.g., by prohibiting imports of plasma from compensated donors) whether this occurs domestically or abroad. The sole ethical argument that could (possibly) justify discriminating between foreign and domestic donors is based on a moral concern for the value of social cohesion. As I outlined in Chapters 6 and 7 one could argue that domestic norms surrounding the procurement of blood and blood products were sufficiently different from those abroad such that while the compensation of donors at home would undermine the cohesiveness of our society it would not have this baleful effect on theirs. A concern for the moral value of social cohesion could thus justify the prohibition of offering compensation to domestic donors while permitting the importation of plasma procured from compensated donors abroad. But (as I argued in Chapters 6 and 7) even the most plausible versions of this argument fail.

Allowing plasma centers to offer compensation to prospective donors is thus required to secure their informed consent, to ensure that the proposals to which they are subject are ones to which they give their authoritative consent, and to avoid their exploitation. Prohibiting compensation thus wrongs donors.

I should also emphasize – *again* – that *prohibiting donor compensation wrongs patients.* As I noted in the Introduction to this volume this debate focuses on *ethics* because the instrumental claims about the effects of compensating plasma donors are settled. The quality of PDMPs produced from plasma secured from compensated donors is no different from those produced from plasma secured from uncompensated donors. And offering donor compensation not only does not decrease the amount of plasma that is procured: It dramatically increases it. Prohibiting plasma centers from offering donor compensation thus decreases the amount of plasma that is available to treat patients. This harms patients. This harm could possibly be justified if the offer of compensation would wrong donors. But it does not. (It is the *prohibition* of compensation that wrongs donors.) Imposing this harm on patients is thus unjustified and wrongful. The prohibition of compensation thus not only wrongs donors: It also harms and wrongs patients.[2]

From Where Should Plasma Be Secured?

These are stark conclusions. But while they are justified with respect to the prohibition of offering compensation to plasma donors, they might not similarly be justified with respect to the prohibition of compensation for the donation of other bodily parts (such as kidneys, corneas, liver lobes, ova, and bone marrow) or services (such as surrogate pregnancy). But before turning to consider the scope of the arguments that I have made in this volume I should in closing address a secondary moral issue associated with the contemporary procurement of plasma: The question of where plasma should be collected.[3]

For the past few decades the WHO has exhorted its member countries to become self-sufficient in blood and blood products.[4] These exhortations have been heeded: Many countries now have self-sufficiency in blood and blood products in general – and plasma in particular – as a stated goal of their healthcare systems.[5] What is striking about this is that despite the almost universal acceptance of self-sufficiency in plasma as a desirable goal there has been almost no philosophical discussion of whether this policy should be pursued.[6] This is unfortunate for pursuing a policy of national self-sufficiency in plasma would for many countries lead to worse healthcare outcomes for their populations given current conditions. This is not because plasma in some countries is generally unsafe, nor is it because some countries could not in principle secure an adequate supply of plasma from within their own borders.[7] (In such cases the WHO encourages the importation of plasma from neighboring countries.)[8] A policy of national self-sufficiency in plasma would *still* be likely to lead to worse healthcare outcomes in a country that pursued this even if its supply was completely safe *and* it could secure enough to meet the medical needs of its population from within its own borders.[9] This is because, for most countries, adopting a policy of self-sufficiency in blood and blood products is more likely to lead to deleterious health outcomes than an alternative approach because this approach to the procurement of blood and blood products would be likely to lead to a wasteful use of limited healthcare resources.

To see why this is so note that the alternative to a country adopting a policy of self-sufficiency in plasma is for it to be willing to import plasma to make up any shortfall in domestic procurement, where the question of whether a shortfall existed would be assessed according to the medical needs of its population.[10] Since a country's ability to import plasma would be (in part) dependent upon another country's ability and willingness to export it, the alternative to countries pursuing policies of self-sufficiency in plasma would be for there to be international trade in it.

Economists have long recognized the advantages of trading over attempting to be self-sufficient.[11] David Ricardo, for example, explained how a country would benefit by producing those goods that it had a lower relative internal opportunity cost to manufacture and then trading these for those goods that other countries could produce at a lower relative internal opportunity cost using the examples of the (then) manufacturing specialties of England and Portugal.[12]

In Ricardo's example, Portugal could produce a certain quantity of wine using the labor of 80 men for one year and a certain quantity of cloth using the labor of 90 men for one year. England could produce the same quantity of cloth using the labor of 100 men for a year and would need to employ 120 men a year to produce the same quantity of wine that Portugal could produce with 80. Given this, it would be to England's benefit to exchange cloth for Portuguese wine. The cloth would cost England the labor of 100 men for a year, but the wine would have cost her the labor of 120 men for a year. England would thus gain from this trade the value of the labor of 20 men for a year. Portugal would also benefit from this, for had she made the cloth that she imported from England herself this would have cost her the value of the labor of 90 men for a year. However, the wine that she traded to get this cloth only cost her the value of the labor of 80 men for a year. Hence, Portugal would gain from this trade the value of the labor of 10 men for a year. Both Portugal and England would lose these gains from trade were they to pursue policies of self-sufficiency with respect to the production of cloth and wine.

Given this economic argument in favor of trade one might infer that for a country to pursue a policy of self-sufficiency in plasma would lead it to forgo the gains that it could garner from participating in an international trade in this good, either as a net exporter of plasma (as is the United States, which allows donor compensation) or as a net importer of it (as is the case for many jurisdictions that prohibit donor compensation). But one might object to this inference by noting that a country's production of plasma is different from its production of goods such as wine and cloth. Unlike these goods, there are no costs (either actual or opportunity) associated with the initial (human) production of plasma. As such, no country has a comparative advantage in the production of plasma over another. Ricardo's argument for the advantage of international trade over national self-sufficiency thus might not apply to plasma for it depends on it being the case that different countries have different comparative advantages in the production of different goods. Since this is not the case for plasma (Scots are not more effective at producing plasma than, say, Italians) the case for international trade that is based on comparative advantage does not apply to it. Any country could thus pursue a policy of self-sufficiency in the production of plasma without forgoing any gains that it could have secured through engaging in an international trade in plasma.

But this objection is misguided. The international trade in plasma is not simply a trade in this good. It is also a trade in the goods and services that are associated with its collection, testing, storage, cataloging, and distribution, as well as a trade in the manufacture, storage, cataloguing, and distribution of the products that are manufactured from source plasma. No country will have a comparative advantage in the (initial, human) production of plasma over any other. But some will have a comparative advantage over others with respect to the provision of the many services associated with the procurement of a safe supply of plasma or with respect to the manufacture of PDMPs.[13] For a country to pursue a policy of self-sufficiency in either plasma or PDMPs when it does not have a comparative advantage in the provision of the services and manufacturing associated with their collection and processing would lead it to forgo the gains that it could secure through participating in international trade in these goods. These gains could have been used to provide additional healthcare for the country's population. Thus, for a country to pursue a policy of national self-sufficiency in plasma when it is not economically advantageous for it to do so would be for it to pursue a health policy that would lead to worse health outcomes for its population than they could have otherwise enjoyed. Hence, if one is concerned about the health of a country's population one should *prima facie* ethically condemn any attempts that it might make to become self-sufficient in plasma or PDMPs if it would be more economically sound for it to import these from elsewhere.[14]

Plasma as a Strategic Resource

The earlier argument treats plasma and PDMPs as though both they and the goods associated with their collection, testing, storage, and so on are goods on a par with wine and cloth. And there's the rub. Unlike wine and cloth, plasma and PDMPs are essential medical supplies. Interruptions to either the ability to procure plasma from donors or to the supply chains involved in both distributing plasma and the manufacture of PDMPs would have serious (and possibly deadly) consequences for the patients that depend on them. The effects of COVID-19 on the world economy have brought these concerns into sharp focus. International supply chains have been seriously disrupted by "restrictions in air transportation facilities, border closure, unavailability of raw material supply, and entire shutdown of manufacturing activities" across multiple industries.[15] Countries that import goods are especially vulnerable to disruptions in their supply chains – whether these are caused by a pandemic or by other shocks such as military action, political disturbance, localized natural disasters, or simply changes in market demand that might cause the needed goods to be diverted into a different geographical area. Biological (or biologically based) medical goods such as plasma and PDMPs are especially vulnerable to interruption in their supply chains. As Paul F.W. Strengers and Harvey G. Klein have noted these supply chains are faced with the risk that "some novel transmissible agent [might] appear" that is "resistant to inactivation or removal technology used in the plasma fractionation industry."[16] If this were to occur in an area that was a leading exporter of plasma those countries that depended upon it for their imports would suffer a severe disruption to their ability to meet the needs of their patients. Moreover, note Strengers and Klein, the supply chains for plasma and PDMPs are also "vulnerable to regulatory actions such as recalls and market withdrawals."[17]

Concerns about possible interruptions to the supply chains for plasma and PDMPs and recognition of the critical importance of these goods for the patients that depend on them led Strengers and Klein to argue that they should be considered strategic resources: "economically important raw materials which are subject to a higher risk of supply interruption."[18] To safeguard access to such resources by guarding against interruptions in their supply chain a country (or region) should strive to become self-sufficient in them. The need to secure the supply of a strategic resource such as plasma or PDMPs could justify the additional costs associated with their procurement and manufacture that would need to be borne by a country that lacks a comparative advantage in these areas when compared with its importation of these goods from a country that possesses such an advantage. To determine if this would be the case, both the risk of disruption to the supply chain and the degree to which this would consequently adversely affect the supply of plasma and PDMPs would need to be assessed.[19] The higher the risk of such disruption and the greater the adverse effect on supply it would cause the higher the costs that a country would be justified in bearing (i.e., by becoming self-sufficient in plasma and PDMPs even if it lacked a comparative advantage in their procurement and manufacture) to avoid this. It is thus possible that a concern for patients could morally justify a country (or region) striving for self-sufficiency in plasma and PDMPs even if it would (currently) be more economically sound for it to import these from elsewhere.

This is a persuasive argument. But the way in which both it and the discussion that preceded it have been framed is misleading. This discussion has addressed the question of whether a country (or region) should strive for self-sufficiency in plasma or PDMPs. In so doing it has moved from questions that concern the justifiability of a *country's* striving for self-sufficiency in these goods to a discussion of whether that *country* would have a comparative advantage in their procurement and manufacture. This is a natural move to make. But it is a misleading one. Ricardo's discussion of comparative advantage addressed the different natural advantages possessed by England and Portugal. (England's climate and soil were well suited for the raising of sheep and the production of cloth, while Portugal's were well suited for growing grapes for making wine.)

In this context, it is natural to ask which country has the comparative advantage in the production of, for example, cloth or wine. But this question is inapt when considering the procurement of plasma and the manufacture of PDMPs. Rather than asking which *country* has the comparative advantage in procuring plasma or manufacturing PDMPs, we should instead ask which *groups of people* have the comparative advantages in these areas. To put this question another way: Which groups of people currently procure plasma and manufacture PDMPs most effectively?

The answer to the part of this question that is the focus of this volume (i.e., which groups of people procure plasma most effectively?) is clear. As Strengers and Klein note, the collection of source plasma in developed countries increased dramatically from 1996 to 2014 with the majority of this increase coming from "the US commercial plasma industry, which historically has dominated international plasma markets."[20] To reinforce the effectiveness of the commercial plasma industry in the United States, Strengers and Klein also note that "[s]ource plasma was collected by 552 commercial plasmapheresis centers of which 80% are located in the United States."[21] Indeed, so successful is the commercial plasma industry in the United States that the plasma it collects "provides not only for the PDMP needs of US patients but also for international export."[22] The groups of people that are most effective at procuring plasma are thus those involved with the commercial procurement of plasma in the United States. And, as noted by Strengers and Klein, the success of the commercial procurement of plasma in the United States is partially dependent upon donor compensation. Thus, the comparative advantage in the procurement of plasma is held by those firms that procure plasma in the United States and that offer compensation to their donors. Together with the arguments in this volume, this data has clear implications for how the future of the global procurement of plasma should unfold: It should primarily be orientated toward the commercial procurement of plasma from compensated donors.

Since the comparative advantage in this industry is possessed by firms rather than by countries or regions, we should now address the question of where these firms should locate their donation centers. It is possible that certain geographic locations might be more attractive to them than others, owing either to the physical infrastructure that is in place or to their regulatory and legal environment. However, even if owing to these differences the costs of procuring plasma would be greater in some areas than others the need to treat plasma and PDMPs as strategic resources could justify their respective procurement and manufacture even in environments that were comparatively *dis*advantaged in these ways. The additional costs that would be incurred could be justified by appeal to the risks (and hence possible costs) associated with not treating plasma and PDMPs as strategic resources and so not striving for self-sufficiency in them. But to ensure that any possible comparative disadvantages are minimized as much as possible the procurement of plasma should be performed by those firms that have the comparative advantage in this. Thus, if it is determined by a country (or region) that the risk of disruption of the supply chains for plasma and PDMPs and the adverse effects associated with this justifies treating these goods as strategic resources, then it should turn to the firms associated with the commercial procurement of plasma to obtain plasma within its borders.

This point is of immediate practical relevance to contemporary healthcare policy. The need efficiently to fractionate plasma has already led some countries (e.g., Finland, Denmark, and Canada) to discontinue fractionating plasma for themselves and contract with commercial firms to do this for them.[23] Other countries (e.g., Australia and France) have followed a similar path, privatizing their state-owned fractionators and then contracting with the private firms that run them to fractionate the blood supply.[24] The use of commercial firms to obtain plasma – and to do so through offering compensating to prospective donors – would not only mitigate the *prima facie* unethical nature of procuring plasma in a situation that is *prima facie* comparatively disadvantageous. It would also address the concerns raised by Strengers and Klein concerning the need to treat plasma and PDMPs as strategic resources. Self-sufficiency could this possibly be ethically justified – but *only* if this approach to procurement is performed efficiently (e.g., by commercial firms) and thereby works to the benefit of patients.

Moving Beyond Plasma: How Far Can the Arguments Extend?

Concern for the well-being of patients should thus support the increasing commercialization of the global plasma supply. This might be a surprising conclusion. But it is less stark than the two primary conclusions that I have reached in this volume: *That the prohibition of donor compensation both harms and wrongs patients, and wrongs donors.* But while these are stark conclusions their scope is limited: It cannot be inferred from the conclusions that prohibiting donor compensation both wrongs and harms patients, and wrongs donors, that the prohibition of offers of compensation for *other* bodily goods and services will also have these adverse effects upon their (potential) recipients and donors.

Plasma is a renewable bodily fluid. The process by which it is extracted from donors is safe, relatively painless, and does not take a lot of time. Source plasma – that which is the focus of this volume – is never transfused directly into patients but instead undergoes extensive processing as the raw material for the manufacture of PDPMs. The donation of plasma thus differs in five important respects from the donation of other bodily parts (such as kidneys, corneas, liver lobes, ova, and bone marrow) or bodily services (such as surrogate pregnancy). First, since source plasma undergoes extensive processing contaminated donations can be identified and excluded. It thus differs from bodily parts (e.g., whole blood) that do not typically undergo such extensive processing before use and whose use, as a result, poses a greater risk to patients. Second, unlike source plasma, some of the other bodily products for whom the question of the morality of donor compensation arises (e.g., kidneys, corneas, and ova) are nonrenewable (although ova are plentiful). Third, unlike, for example, surrogate pregnancy or kidney donation the donation of plasma is unlikely to impose any psychological costs on the donor.[25] Fourth, the process by which other donated bodily parts are extracted is more dangerous, painful, or time-consuming than the donation of plasma.[26] These considerations also distinguish the donation of plasma from surrogate pregnancy. Not only is pregnancy (obviously) far more time-consuming than donating plasma it is also more physically dangerous.[27] Finally, the latter two differences between the provision of plasma and the provision of other bodily parts and services are reflected in the level of compensation that would be offered for them. The typical plasma donor in the United States receives just $35 for a donation.[28] By contrast, a person who carries, for example, a surrogate pregnancy to term in the United States receives on average $23,000.[29]

These empirical differences between plasma on the one hand and other bodily parts and services on the other may lead to moral differences with respect to the permissibility of offering compensation for their provision.[30]

First, the processing that source plasma undergoes during its manufacture into PDMPs has moral import. As a result of this processing – and as I have extensively documented in this volume – PDMPs manufactured from plasma secured from compensated donors pose no more risk to patients than do PDMPs manufactured from plasma secured from uncompensated donors. However, safety concerns might still be relevant to discussions of the use of compensation to encourage donors to donate *other* body parts that do not undergo such extensive processing before use, and so are more likely to transmit infectious agents. Titmuss-style arguments concerning the adverse selection effects of compensated donations might thus apply to the debates over whether the donors of other bodily products (such as whole blood) should be compensated even though they do not (currently) apply to the debate over whether plasma donors should be compensated.[31]

Second, the distinction between the renewability of plasma and the nonrenewability of other bodily products could also be relevant to the question of whether or not it is morally permissible to procure them by offering compensation to their prospective donors. Kant, for example, objects to both the sale and the donation of "an organ of the body" while allowing that it would be permissible (if "not altogether free of blame") to remove for sale something that was "a part but not an organ of the body."[32] For Kant, then, while kidney donation (whether compensated or uncompensated) would be morally impermissible offering compensation for plasma donors *might* be permissible – depending on whether plasma is considered to be "an organ of the body" or not.[33]

Third, the different psychological effects that plasma donation and the donation of other bodily parts or services are likely to have on the donor will be morally relevant. The psychological costs associated with surrogate pregnancy, for example, were drawn upon by Elizabeth Anderson to object to this practice. Anderson objects to surrogacy contracts – whether compensated or uncompensated – on the deontic grounds that they will treat "the mother's inalienable right to love her child, and to express that love by asserting a claim to custody in its own best interests, as if it were alienable in a market transaction."[34] This is wrongful, Anderson argues, because a mother's right to love her child is not grounded in the mother's interests but in the obligations that she has to her child. In requiring a mother emotionally to distance herself from her child a surrogacy contract will require the mother to fail to fulfill her duty to her. Drawing on Kant's conception of autonomy (on which persons act autonomously not by pursuing their "optional personal projects" but by fulfilling their duties) Anderson holds that requiring a mother to fail to fulfill her duty to the child will thereby compromise her autonomy.[35] Thus, for Anderson, surrogacy is inherently wrongful because it inherently fails to respect the autonomy of the mother.[36] But the duties that render surrogacy wrongful for Anderson are not at issue when considering the morality of plasma donation. Both Kant and Anderson might thus accept that the arguments in this volume establish that donor compensation is not only permissible but morally required out of concern for both donors and patients. Doing so would not commit them to holding that the compensated (or uncompensated) donation of other bodily parts or services is also thereby morally justified.

The fourth distinction between the donation of plasma and the provision of other bodily parts or services (that the latter are more dangerous, painful, or time-consuming than the former) is also morally relevant. It is plausible to hold that the riskier an activity is the more justified one would be in paternalistically prohibiting it – whether this be justified on deontic or consequentialist grounds. Since, for example, pregnancy, nephrectomy, and ovarian stimulation are all riskier activities than plasma donation, a paternalist would be more justified in prohibiting compensated surrogate pregnancy, or compensation for donation of kidneys or ova, than she would be justified in prohibiting compensated plasma donation.[37]

This distinction could also ground an argument for the conclusion that while it is morally permissible to offer compensation to prospective plasma donors, in some situations it would be morally *im*permissible to offer compensation to prospective kidney donors. Recall (from Chapter 3) that for an offer to be permissible two conditions must be met:

(1) Given the situation that they are in both parties would be autonomous with respect to their preference that the proposed token exchange take place rather than not and (2) both parties would be autonomous with respect to their preference that exchanges of that type are allowed rather than precluded, as both believe that allowing them could lead to an increase in their respective well-being.[38] It is likely that both those who operate plasma centers that are willing to compensate their donors and prospective plasma donors would meet both of these conditions with respect to offers of compensation for donation. But it is much less likely that condition (2) would always be met by prospective kidney donors. In some developing countries, there is a significant gender imbalance in kidney donation with women donating at a far higher rate than men.[39] It is thus likely that were those countries to allow compensation for kidney donation this imbalance would be replicated in the realm of compensated kidney donation. It is accordingly possible that many of those (i.e., women) who would donate their kidneys for compensation were this to be allowed would recognize that this imbalance would occur and would accordingly prefer that exchanges of this type continue to be prohibited.[40] And they would prefer that such exchanges be prohibited because they recognize that they would be subject to harm (i.e., that associated with the donation of their kidney) if they were to be allowed and they all things considered wish to avoid this.

Finally, the differing levels of compensation that would be offered for plasma and for other bodily goods or services will also be morally relevant. It is, for example, possible that prospective kidney donors might have less need than prospective plasma donors to know the economic value of their donations before they could give their informed consent to donate. Even absent this information a prospective kidney donor would realize that her donation had an economic value that was likely to be greater than her opportunity costs of donating. Individual plasma donations, however, have relatively low economic value. It is thus more likely that a prospective plasma donor's opportunity costs would exceed the economic value of their donation than those of a prospective kidney donor would exceed theirs. The provision of information concerning the precise economic value of their donations would thus (all things being equal) be more relevant to prospective plasma donors than to prospective kidney donors. The moral concern with securing donor's informed consent (that grounded the arguments in Chapter 2) is thus more likely to support the need to offer compensation to plasma donors than it is to support the need to offer this to kidney donors.

Finis

The arguments in this volume that support the moral imperative to offer compensation to prospective plasma donors might thus not translate into similarly supporting the need to offer compensation to the donors of other bodily parts or services. But this limitation in the scope of these arguments is a positive feature rather than a drawback. It shows that they are responsive to those aspects of the world that are relevant to them rather than simply imposing a view of morality upon it. Given the force of the arguments in this volume, I hope that those involved in determining whether donor compensation should be allowed or prohibited are similarly responsive to those features of the world that should be relevant to their decisions – such as moral argument. If they are not, then the bioethics that would be drawn upon (putatively) to support prohibiting donor compensation for plasma will be bloody indeed.

Notes

1. A version of this paragraph appeared in James Stacey Taylor, "Why Prohibiting Donor Compensation Can Prevent Plasma Donors from Giving Their Informed Consent to Donate," *Journal of Medicine and Philosophy* 44, 1 (2019), 10.
2. It also wrongs those who would operate plasma centers that would offer compensation to their donors.
3. An earlier version of this discussion appeared in James Stacey Taylor, "Why Policies that Aim at National Self-Sufficiency in Blood and Blood Products are (Usually) Unethical," *Public Affairs Quarterly* 29, 3 (2015), 313–326.
4. WHO, *Towards Self-Sufficiency in Safe Blood and Blood Products*, 2. (For a discussion of this document see Taylor, "A Scandal in Geneva.") See, too, the WHO Expert Group, "Expert Consensus Statement on Achieving Self-Sufficiency in Safe Blood and Blood Products, Based on Voluntary Non-Remunerated Blood Donation (VNRBD)," *Vox Sanguinis* 103, 4 (2012), 337–342. See also the WHO, "The Rome Declaration on Achieving Self-Sufficiency in Safe Blood and Blood Products, based on Voluntary Non-Remunerated Donation," Available at: www.avis.it/userfiles/file/RomeDeclarationSelf-SufficiencySafeBloodBloodProductsVNRD.pdf; and the "Sixty-Third World Health Assembly, Resolution WHA63.12," Available at: http://apps.who.int/gb/ebwha/pdf_files/WHA63/A63_R12-en.pdf (The WHA is the decision-making body of the WHO). The authors of the *Rome Declaration* held that *The Melbourne Declaration on 100% Voluntary Non-Remunerated Donation of Blood and Blood Components* (June 2009) and WHA Resolutions WHA28.72 (www.who.int/bloodsafety/en/WHA28.72.pdf), WHA56.30 (www.who.int/3by5/en/WHA03AIDS.pdf), WHA58.13 (http://apps.who.int/iris/bitstream/10665/20363/1/WHA58_13-en.pdf) "have reaffirmed the achievement of self-sufficiency in blood and blood products based on voluntary non-remunerated blood donation (VNRBD) as the important national policy direction for ensuring a safe, secure and sufficient supply of blood and blood products" (p. 3). This claim is false. None of these documents address this issue at all.
5. In Italy, for example, "the achievement of self-sufficiency of plasma-derived medicinal products . . . is a goal of the blood system" See Gabriele Calizzani et al., "Plasma and Plasma-Derived Medicinal Product Self-Sufficiency: The Italian Case," *Blood Transfusion* 11, Suppl. 4 (2013), s118. Doubts about the practicality of such a policy for Italy are expressed by Vincenzo de Angelis and Antonio Breda, "Plasma-Derived Medicinal Products Self-Sufficiency

From National Plasma: To What Extent?," *Blood Transfusion* 11, Suppl. 4 (2013), 132–137. In France, part of the mission of the EFS is "guaranteeing national self-sufficiency in blood products." (Françoise Rossi, "The Organization of Transfusion and Fractionation in France and Its Regulation," *Annals of Blood* 3 (2018). Available at: http://aob.amegroups.com/article/view/4610/5358. That Spain has a goal of becoming self-sufficient in plasma (as much as possible) is noted by Rovira, "Plasma Self-sufficiency in Spain." The National Blood Authority of Australia states that "Australia is committed to being self-sufficient in its supply of blood and blood products where feasible." National Blood Authority, "Why Does Australia Import Blood Products?" Available at: www.blood.gov.au/imported-products

6. Although see Taylor, "Why Policies that Aim at National Self-Sufficiency in Blood and Blood Products are (Usually) Unethical," and Flanagan, "Self-Sufficiency in Plasma Supply – Achievable and Desirable?" 483–487.

7. The Government of the United Kingdom recently lifted the ban on using UK-sourced plasma for the manufacture of immunoglobulins, a ban that was enacted in 1998 as a result of concerns about the contamination of British blood and blood products by Creutzfeldt Jakob Disease. See Department of Health and Social Care, "Ban Lifted to Allow UK Blood Plasma to be Used for Life-Saving Treatments," (February 25, 2021). Available at: www.gov.uk/government/news/ban-lifted-to-allow-uk-blood-plasma-to-be-used-for-life-saving-treatments

8. WHO, *Towards Self-Sufficiency in Safe Blood and Blood Products*, 2.

9. Although such self-sufficiency is unlikely for many countries; see de Angelis and Breda, "Plasma-Derived Medicinal Products Self-Sufficiency from National Plasma: To What Extent?" 137.

10. See the related discussion in Chapters 6 and 7.

11. See, for example, Adam Smith, *An Inquiry into the Nature and Causes of the Wealth of Nations* (Chicago: University of Chicago Press, 1976), 478–479.

12. David Ricardo, *On the Principles of Political Economy and Taxation* (London: J. M. Dent & Sons, 1911), Chapter 7.

13. A country such as the United States, for example, which has an established commercial industry devoted to procuring source plasma and manufacturing PDMPs will have a comparative advantage over a country that lacks this owing to both efficiencies of scale and its possession of established infrastructure.

14. I did not originally realize that the conclusion of this argument should only be a *prima facia* condemnation of such a move to self-sufficiency for I did not initially recognize the possible importance of plasma and PDMPs as strategic resources. My original conclusion was thus too strong. See Taylor, "Why Policies that Aim at National Self-Sufficiency in Blood and Blood Products are (Usually) Unethical," 313–326.

15. Kazi Safowan Shahed, Abdullahil Azeem, Syed Mithun Ali, and Md. Abdul Moktadir, "A Supply Chain Disruption Risk Mitigation Model to Manage COVID-19 Pandemic Risk," *Environmental Science and Pollution Research* (January 15, 2021), 1. Available at: https://doi.org/10.1007/s11356-020-12289-4.

16. Strengers and Klein, "Plasma is a Strategic Resource," 3135. See also Albert Farrugia and Daniela Scaramuccia, "The Dynamics of Contract Plasma Fractionation," *Biologicals* 46 (2017), 162, and Rovira, "Plasma Self-Sufficiency in Spain," 2.

17. Strengers and Klein, "Plasma is a Strategic Resource," 3135.

18. Ibid. Strengers and Klein claim that this is the definition of strategic goods offered by the European Union. However, they do not cite any documents

from an EU body in support of this claim but instead cite a document from the British Government's Department of Environment, Food, and Rural Affairs, *A Review of National Resource Strategies and Research* (London: H.M. Government, 2012), 1, that focuses on the strategic importance of rare earths. This document in turn cites an EU document which is putatively located at: http://ec.europa.eu/enterprise/policies/raw-materials/criti cal/index_en.htm However, this document no longer exists. Moreover, no EU document that defines strategic resource in the way accepted as the EU definition by Strengers and Klein exists. This does not, however, make a difference to this argument for nothing rests on this definition.

19. Strengers and Klein do not address these issues, wrongly assuming that self-sufficiency to guard against supply interruptions would always be justified.

20. Strengers and Klein, "Plasma is a Strategic Resource," 3134.

21. Ibid.

22. Ibid.

23. Farrugia and Scaramuccia, "The Dynamics of Contract Plasma Fractionation." Note that the claim is not that all state-run fractionation has been discontinued in these countries.

24. Ibid.

25. For an overview of the psychological costs borne by surrogate mothers see Hoda Ahmari Tehran, Shohreh Tashi, Nahid Mehran, Narges Eskandari, and Tahmineh Dadkhah Tehrani, "Emotional Experiences in Surrogate Mothers: A Qualitative Study," *Iranian Journal of Reproductive Medicine* 12, 7 (2014), 471–480. For an overview of the psychological costs associated with the compensated donation of a kidney see Julian Koplin, "Assessing the Likely Harms to Kidney Vendors in Regulated Organ Markets," *The American Journal of Bioethics* 14, 10 (2014), 7–18.

26. Semen donation is the obvious exception here. The risks involved in nephrectomy are outlined in Taylor, *Stakes and Kidneys*, 125–130. The risks involved in ova donation are outlined in Amy E. White, "The Morality of an Internet Market in Human Ova," *Journal of Value Inquiry* 40 (2006), 313–314.

27. See, for example, Snigdha Reddy and Belinda Jim, "Hypertension and Pregnancy: Management and Future Risks," *Advances in Chronic Kidney Disease* 26, 2 (2019), 137–145; Andrea G. Kattah and Vesna D. Garovic, "Preeclampsia: Cardiovascular and Renal Risks During and After Pregnancy," in Babbett LaMarca and Barbara T. Alexander, eds., *Sex Differences in Cardiovascular Physiology and Pathophysiology* (London: Academic Press, 2019), 137–147.

28. Skinner et al., "Risk-Based Decision Making and Ethical Considerations in Donor Compensation for Plasma-Derived Medicinal Products," 2891.

29. Hillary L. Berk, "Savvy Surrogates and Rock Star Parents: Compensation Provisions, Contracting Practices, and the Value of Womb Work," *Law & Social Inquiry* 45, 2 (2020), 409.

30. For a discussion of how differences between different body parts might justify allowing compensation to be offered for some but not for others see Erik Malmqvist, "Does the Ethical Appropriateness of Paying Donors Depend on What Body Parts They Donate?" *Medicine, Health Care, and Philosophy* 19 (2016), 463–473.

31. Jeremy Shearmur, "Trust, Titmuss, and Blood," *Economic Affairs* 21, 1 (2001), 29. The caveat "currently" is included to recognize that it is possible that in the future an infectious agent might appear that is both associated with populations of compensated donors are that cannot be detected or eliminated by current processing methods.

32. Immanuel Kant, *The Metaphysics of Morals*, M. Gregor, trans. (Cambridge: Cambridge University Press, 1991), 219.
33. Kant's argument is criticized in Taylor, *Stakes and Kidneys*, 153–155. Other Kantian arguments against organ sale are addressed in Cherry, *Kidney for Sale By Owner*, 133–137.
34. Elizabeth S. Anderson, "Why Commercial Surrogate Motherhood Unethically Commodifies Women and Children: Reply to McLachlan and Swales," *Health Care Analysis* 8 (2000), 23. Brennan and Jaworski mischaracterize Anderson's position as one where it is morally permissible to serve as a surrogate for free but not for pay. (*Markets Without Limits*, 12.) This is not Anderson's view. See Taylor, *Markets with Limits*, Chapter 4.
35. Ibid., 23.
36. Ibid., 23–24.
37. She would also be more justified in prohibiting uncompensated surrogate pregnancy or the donation of kidneys or ova than she would be justified in prohibiting uncompensated plasma donation.
38. See Taylor, "How Not to Argue for Markets," 165–179.
39. M.M. Bal and B. Saikia "Gender Bias in Renal Transplantation: Are Women Alone Donating Kidneys in India?" *Transplantation Proceedings* 39, 10 (2007), 2961–2963. This point can also be made with respect to bonded laborers. See Syed Ali Anwar Naqvi, Bux Ali, Farida Mazhar, Mirza Naqi Zafar, and Syed Adibul Hasan Rizvi, A Socioeconomic Survey of Kidney Vendors in Pakistan," *Transplant International* 20, 11 (2007), 934–939. See also Sigrid Fry-Revere, Deborah Chen, Bahar Bastani, Simin Golestani, Rachana Agarwal, Howsikan Kugathasan, and Melissa Le, "Coercion, Dissatisfaction, and Social Stigma: An Ethnographic Study of Compensated Living Kidney Donation in Iran," *International Urology and Nephrology* 52 (2020), 2403–2414.
40. Note that the conclusion of this speculative argument is not that kidney sales would be morally wrong, but that they would be morally wrong in certain circumstances.

Bibliography

Adams, Vincanne, Kathleen Erwin, and Phuoc V. Le, "Public Health Works: Blood Donation in Urban China," *Social Science & Medicine* 68 (2009): 410–418.

Adashek, Eugene P., and William H. Adashek, "Blood-Transfusion Hepatitis in Open-Heart Surgery," *Archives of Surgery* 87, 5 (1963): 792–795.

Allain, J-P., "Volunteer Safer Than Replacement Donor Blood: A Myth Revealed by Evidence," *ISBT Science Series* 5, 1 (2010): 169–175.

Ambuehl, Sandro, Axel Ockenfels, and Alvin E. Roth, "Payment in Challenge Studies from an Economics Perspective," *BMJ Journal of Medical Ethics* 46, 12 (2020): 831–832.

Anderson, Benedict, *Imagined Communities: Reflections on the Origin and Spread of Nationalism* (London: Verso, 1983).

Anderson, Elizabeth S., "Why Commercial Surrogate Motherhood Unethically Commodifies Women and Children: Reply to McLachlan and Swales," *Health Care Analysis* 8 (2000): 19–26.

Archard, David, "Selling Yourself: Titmuss's Argument Against a Market in Blood," *Journal of Ethics* 6, 1 (2002): 87–103.

Arrow, Kenneth J., "Gifts and Exchanges," *Philosophy & Public Affairs* 1, 4 (1972): 343–362.

Aspinall, Butler, ed., *Reports of Cases Relating to Maritime Law Containing All the Decisions of The Courts of Law and Equity in The United Kingdom* (London, Horace Cox, 1905, vol. 9).

Bal, M.M., and B. Saikia, "Gender Bias in Renal Transplantation: Are Women Alone Donating Kidneys in India?" *Transplantation Proceedings* 39, 10 (2007): 2961–2963.

Beal, R.W., and W.G. van Aken, "Gift or Good? A Contemporary Examination of the Voluntary and Commercial Aspects of Blood Donation," *Vox Sanguinis* 63, 1 (1992): 1–5.

Beauchamp, Tom L., "Who Deserves Autonomy, and Whose Autonomy Deserves Respect," in James Stacey Taylor, ed., *Personal Autonomy: New Essays on Personal Autonomy and Its Role in Contemporary Moral Philosophy* (Cambridge: Cambridge University Press, 2005): 310–329.

Beauchamp, Tom L., and James F. Childress, *Principles of Biomedical Ethics* (New York: Oxford University Press, 2013, 7th edn).

Bechtloff, S., B. Tran-My, H. Haubelt, G. Stelzer, C. Anders, and P. Hellstern, "A Prospective Trial on the Safety of Long-Term Intensive Plasmapheresis in Donors," *Vox Sanguinis* 88 (2005): 189–195.

Berk, Hillary R., "Savvy Surrogates and Rock Star Parents: Compensation Provisions, Contracting Practices, and the Value of Womb Work," *Law & Social Inquiry* 45, 2 (2020): 398–431.

Berntrop, Erik, and Amy D. Shapiro, "Modern Hemophilia Care," *The Lancet* 379, 9824 (2012): 1447–1456.

Bharati, K. Pavani, and U. Ram Prashanth, "Von Willebrand Disease: An Overview," *Indian Journal of Pharmaceutical Sciences* 73, 1 (2011): 7–16.

Bloch, Evan M., et al., "Deployment of Convalescent Plasma for the Prevention and Treatment of COVID-19," *Journal of Clinical Investigation* 130, 6 (2020): 2757–2765.

Bloodwatch, "Securing & Protecting The Canadian Blood Supply Why We Need A Legislative Ban on Paid-Plasma in Canada Senate of Canada & House of Commons Brief," (October 2018).

Borgstrom, Erica, Simon Cohn, and Stephen Barclay, "Medical Professionalism: Conflicting Values for Tomorrow's Doctors," *Journal of General Internal Medicine* 25, 12 (2010): 1330–1336.

Bove, Liliana L., Tim Bednall, Barbara Masser, and Mark Buzza, "Understanding the Plasmapheresis Donor in a Voluntary, Nonremunerated Environment," *Transfusion* 51 (2011): 2411–2424.

Bowles, Samuel, and Sandra Polanía-Reyes, "Economic Incentives and Social Preferences: Substitutes or Complements?" *Journal of Economic Literature* 50, 2 (2012): 368–425.

B-Positive, "Donate Plasma, Get Paid, Save Lives," Available at: www.bpositivetoday.com/

Brennan, Jason, and Peter M. Jaworski, *Markets Without Limits: Moral Virtues and Commercial Interests* (New York: Routledge: 2016).

Brink, David O., "Retributivism and Legal Moralism," *Ratio Juris* 25, 4 (2012): 496–512.

British Government Department of Environment, Food, and Rural Affairs, *A Review of National Resource Strategies and Research* (London: H.M. Government, 2012).

Brown, Jerry F., Kathleen Rowe, Peter Zacharias, James van Hasselt, John M. Dye, David A. Wohl, William A. Fischer Nd, Coleen K. Cunningham, Nathan M. Thielman, and David L. Hoover, "Apheresis for Collection of Ebola Convalescent Plasma in Liberia," *Journal of Clinical Apheresis* 32, 3 (2017): 175–181.

Burnouf, Thierry, "Modern Plasma Fractionation," *Transfusion Medicine Reviews* 21, 2 (2007): 101–117.

Burnouf, Thierry, "An Overview of Plasma Fractionation," *Annals of Blood* 3, 33 (2018): 1–10.

Buyx, Alena M., "Blood Donation, Payment, and Non-Cash Incentives: Classical Questions Drawing Renewed Interest," *Transfusion medicine and hemotherapy: offizielles Organ der Deutschen Gesellschaft fur Transfusionsmedizin und Immunhamatologie* 36, 5 (2009): 330–331.

Calizzani, Gabriele, S. Profili, F. Candursa, M. Lanzoni, S. Vaglio, L. Cannata, L. Catalano, R. Chianese, G.M. Liumbruno, and G. Grazzini, "Plasma and Plasma-Derived Medicinal Product Self-Sufficiency: The Italian Case," *Blood Transfusion* 11, Suppl. 4 (2013): s118–s131.

Campbell, Alastair V., *The Body in Bioethics* (New York: Routledge-Cavendish, 2009).

Campbell, Alastair V., Cecilia Tan, and F. Elias Boujaoude, "The Ethics of Blood Donation: Does Altruism Suffice?" *Biologicals* 40, 3 (2012): 170–172.

Canadian Blood Services, "Our Commitment to Increasing Plasma Sufficiency in Canada," Available at: https://blood.ca/en/about-us/media/plasma/plasma-sufficiency

Canadian Health Coalition, "Unpaid Plasma and Blood Donation," Available at: www.healthcoalition.ca/unpaid-plasma-and-blood-donations/

Canadian Nurses Association, "Resolution 4: Protect Canada's Blood Supply by Rejecting For-Profit Plasma Collection," Available at: https://rnao.ca/sites/rnao-ca/files/Resolution_4_-_Protect_Canadas_Blood_Supply_by_Rejecting_for-Profit_Plasma_Collection.pdf

Canturbury v. Spence 464 F .2d 772 (D.C. Cir. 1972).

Carroll, Lewis, *Through the Looking-Glass, and What Alice Found There* (London: Macmillan & Co., 1872).

Charbonneau, Johanne, Marie-Soleil Cloutier, and Élianne Carrier, "Whole Blood and Apheresis Donors in Quebec, Canada: Demographic Differences and Motivations to Donate," *Transfusion and Apheresis Science* 53, 3 (2015): 320–328.

Charities Aid Foundation, *CAF World Giving Index 2019* (West Malling, Kent: Charities Aid Foundation, 2019).

Chell, Kathleen, Tanya E. Davison, Barbara Masser, and Kyle Jensen, "A Systematic Review of Incentives in Blood Donation," *Transfusion* 58 (2018): 242–254.

Cherry, Mark J., *Kidney for Sale By Owner* (Washington, DC: Georgetown University Press, 2005).

Cherry, Mark J., and Ruiping Fan, "Informed Consent: The Decisional Standing of Families," *Journal of Medicine and Philosophy* 40 (2015): 363–370.

Cherry, Mark J., and H. Tristram Engelhardt, Jr., "Informed Consent in Texas: Theory and Practice," *Journal of Medicine and Philosophy* 29, 2 (2004): 237–252.

CSL Plasma, "Coupon Offer," Available at: www.cslplasma.com/center/NJ/199-hamilton/coupon?gclid=EAIaIQobChMIg8WZ9Zn55gIVCaGzCh2-zgwAEAMYASAAEgL4v_D_BwE

de Angelis, Vincenzo, and Antonio Breda, "Plasma-Derived Medicinal Products Self-Sufficiency from National Plasma: To What Extent?," *Blood Transfusion* 11, Suppl. 4 (2013): 132–137.

Delhey, Jan, and Kenneth Newton, "Predicting Cross-National Levels of Social Trust: Global Pattern or Nordic Exceptionalism?" *European Sociological Review* 21, 4 (2005): 311–327.

del Pozo, Pablo Rodriguez, "Paying Donors and the Ethics of Blood Supply," *Journal of Medical Ethics* 20 (1994): 31–35.

Del Prete, F., "A Study of the IP Factor in Blood Donors," *Presented at the Sixth Annual Meeting of the South Central Association of Blood Banks, Oklahoma City* (March 1964).

De Silvestro, Giustina, Piero Marson, Antonio Breda, and Vincenz De Angelis, "Plasma-Derived Industry and Plasma-Derived Medicinal Products in the

Italian National Blood Transfusion Service," *Transfusion and Apheresis Science* 58, 5 (2019): 545–549.

Dougherty, W.J., "Narcotics Associated Hepatitis – New Jersey," *Morbidity and Mortality Weekly Report* 16, 21 (1967): 170.

Dowie, Mark, "Pinto Madness," *Mother Jones* (September/October 1977). Available at: www.motherjones.com/politics/1977/09/pinto-madness/

Dworkin, Gerald, "Acting Freely," *Nous* 4, 4 (1970): 367–383.

Dworkin, Gerald, "Markets and Morals: The Case for Organ Sales," in Gerald Dworkin, ed., *Morality, Harm, and the Law* (Boulder, CO: Westview Press, 1994): 155–161.

Ekstrom, Laura Waddell, "Autonomy and Personal Integration," in James Stacey Taylor, ed., *Personal Autonomy: New Essays on Personal Autonomy and Its Role in Contemporary Moral Philosophy* (Cambridge: Cambridge University Press, 2005): 143–161.

Erwin, Kathleen, "The Circulatory System: Blood Procurement, AIDS, and the Social Body in China," *Medical Anthropology Quarterly* 20, 2 (2006): 139–159.

Etablissement français du sang, "Le don de plasma," Available at: https://donde-sang.efs.sante.fr/le-don-de-plasma

Etablissement français du sang, "Missing Type," Available at: https://missing-type.efs.sante.fr/

European Agency for the Evaluation of Medicinal Products, "CPMP Position Statement Non-Remunerated and Remunerated Donors: Safety and Supply of Plasma-Derived Medicinal Products," (May 30, 2002).

European Commission Directorate-General for Health and Food Safety, "Summary Minutes of a Meeting between CSL, PPTA, and DG SANTE P4," (January 21, 2016). Available at: https://ec.europa.eu/health/sites/health/files/blood_tissues_organs/docs/ares20166855155_summary_minutes.pdf

Faden, Ruth R., Tom L. Beauchamp, and Nancy M.P. King, *A History and Theory of Informed Consent* (New York: Oxford University Press, 1986).

Farrell, Anne-Maree, *The Politics of Blood: Ethics, Innovation, and the Regulation of Risk* (Cambridge: Cambridge University Press, 2012).

Farrugia, A., and C. Del Bo, "Some reflections on the Code of Ethics of the International Society of Blood Transfusion," *Blood Transfusion* 13, 4 (2015): 551–558.

Farrugia, A., J. Penrod, and J.M. Bult, "Payment, Compensation and Replacement – the Ethics and Motivation of Blood and Plasma Donation," *Vox Sanguinis* 60, S3 (2010): 202–211.

Farrugia, A., J. Penrod, and J.M. Bult, "The Ethics of Paid Plasma Donation: A Plea for Patient Centeredness," *HEC Forum* 27 (2015): 426.

Ferguson, E., K. Farrell, and C. Lawrence, "Blood Donation is an Act of Benevolence Rather than Altruism," *Health Psychology* 27, 3 (2008): 327–336.

Fildes, Valerie, "The English Wet-Nurse and Her Role in Infant Care 1538–1800," *Medical History* 32 (1988): 142–173.

Flanagan, Peter, "The Code of Ethics of the International Society of Blood Transfusion," *Blood Transfusion* 13, 4 (2015): 537–538.

Flanagan, Peter, "Self-Sufficiency in Plasma Supply – Achievable and Desirable?" *ISBT Science Series* 12 (2017): 483–487.

Flynn v. Holder, "United States Court of Appeals for the Ninth Circuit," (December 1, 2011).

Folléa, Grilles, Erhard Seifried, and Jeroen de Wit, "Renewed Considerations on Ethical Values for Blood and Plasma Donations and Donors," *Blood Transfusion* 12, Suppl. 1 (2014): s387–s388.

Fontaine, Richard, "Richard Titmuss on Social Cohesion: A Comment," *European Journal of Political Economy* 20 (2004): 795–797.

Food and Drug Administration, "Volume Limits – Automated Collection of Source Plasma," (November 4, 1992).

Food and Drug Administration Center for Biologics Evaluation and Research, "Blood Products Advisory Committee Meeting, Transcript Prepared by CASET Associates Ltd," (April 28, 2011).

Frankfurt, Harry G., "Freedom of the Will and the Concept of a Person," *The Journal of Philosophy* 68, 1 (1971): 5–20.

Frankfurt, Harry G., "Autonomy, Necessity, and Love," in Harry G. Frankfurt, ed., *Necessity, Volition, and Love* (Cambridge: Cambridge University Press, 1998): 129–141.

Freiman, Christopher, "Vote Markets," *Australasian Journal of Philosophy* 92, 4 (2014): 759–774.

Friedman, Michael A., "Testimony on the GAO Report on 'Blood Plasma Safety,'" (September 9, 1998). Available at: www.hhs.gov/asl/testify/t980909a.html

Fry-Revere, Sigrid, Deborah Chen, Bahar Bastani, Simin Golestani, Rachana Agarwal, Howsikan Kugathasan, and Melissa Le, "Coercion, Dissatisfaction, and Social Stigma: An Ethnographic Study of Compensated Living Kidney Donation in Iran," *International Urology and Nephrology* 52 (2020): 2403–2414.

Geha, Raif S., et al., "Primary Immunodeficiency Diseases: An Update from the International Union of Immunological Societies Primary Immunodeficiency Diseases Classification Committee," *Journal of Allergy and Clinical Immunology* 120, 4 (2007): 776–794.

George, Rose, *Nine Pints; A Journey Through the Money, Medicine, and Mysteries of Blood* (New York: Metropolitan Books, 2018).

Gillon, R., "Ethics Needs Principles – Four Can Encompass the Rest – and Respect for Autonomy Should be 'First Among Equals'" *Journal of Medical Ethics* 29 (2003): 307–312.

Gneezy, Uri, Stephan Meier, and Pedro Rey-Biel, "When and Why Incentives (Don't) Work to Modify Behavior," *Journal of Economic Perspectives* 25, 4 (Fall 2011): 191–210.

Gneezy, Uri, and Aldo Rustichini, "A Fine is a Price," *Journal of Legal Studies* 29, 1 (2000): 1–17.

Gneezy, Uri, and Aldo Rustichini, "Pay Enough – or Don't Pay at All," *The Quarterly Journal of Economics* 115, 3 (2000): 791–810.

Government of Canada, "Backgrounder Paper – Plasma Donations in Canada," Available at: www.canada.ca/en/health-canada/services/drugs-health-products/public-involvement-consultations/biologics-radiopharmaceuticals-genetic-therapies/backgrounder-paper-plasma-donations-canada.html

Grabowski, Henry G., and Richard L. Manning, "An Economic Analysis of Global Policy Proposals to Prohibit Compensation of Blood Plasma Donors," *International Journal of the Economics of Business* 23, 2 (2016): 149–166.

Grady, George F., Thomas C. Chalmers, and The Boston Inter-Hospital Liver Group, "Risk of Post-Transfusion Viral hepatitis," *New England Journal of Medicine* 271, 7 (1964): 337–342.

Grainger, Brian, and Peter Flanagan, "Informed Consent for Whole Blood Donation," *Vox Sanguinis* 115, 1 (2020): 3–10.

Grazzini, Giuliano, Pier Mannuccio, and Fabrizio Oleari, "Plasma Derived Medicinal Products: Demand and Clinical Use," *Blood Transfusion* 11, Suppl. 4 (2013): S2–S5.

Grifols, "Buddy Bonus Program," Available at: www.grifolsplasma.com/en/returning-plasma-donors/buddy-bonus-program

Grifols, "How to Donate Plasma," Available at: www.grifolsplasma.com/en/plasma-donor/how-to-donate/donation-fees

Grifols, V., "Financing Plasma Proteins: Unique Challenges," *Pharmaceutical Policy and Law* 7 (2006): 185–198.

Hagen, Piet J., *Blood Transfusion in Europe: A "White Paper"* (Strasbourg: Council of Europe Press, 1993).

Hansen-Magnusson, Hannes, "Governance in the European Union: The European Blood Directive as an Evolving Practice," *Clinics in Laboratory Medicine* 30, 2 (2010): 489–497.

Hartmann, Jan, and Harvey G. Klein, "Supply and Demand for Plasma-Derived Medicinal Products - A Critical Reassessment Amid the COVID-19 Pandemic," *Transfusion* 60, 11 (2020): 2748–2752.

Hausman, Jerry, and Ephraim Leibtag, "Consumer Benefits from Increased Competition in Shopping Outlets: Measuring the Effect of Wal-Mart," *Journal of Applied Econometrics* 22 (2007): 1157–1177.

Health Canada, *Protecting Access to Immune Globulins for Canadians. Final report of the Expert Panel on the Immune Globulin Product Supply and Related Impacts in Canada* (Ottawa: Health Canada, 2018).

Healy, Kieran, *Last Best Gifts: Altruism and the Market for Human Blood and Organs* (Chicago: University of Chicago Press, 2006).

Hema-Quebec, "Annual Report 2013–2014," Available at: www.hema-quebec.qc.ca/userfiles/file/RA_2013-2014/HQ_RA_2013-2014_ANG_FINAL(1).pdf

Hema-Quebec, "Annual Report 2014–2015," Available at: www.hema-quebec.qc.ca/userfiles/file/media/anglais/publications/RA_2014-2015_ANG(2).pdf

Hema-Quebec, "Annual Report 2015–2016," Available at: www.hema-quebec.qc.ca/userfiles/file/RA-2015-2016/RA_2015-2016_ANG-2.pdf

Hema-Quebec, "Annual Report 2016–2017," Available at: www.hema-quebec.qc.ca/userfiles/file/media/anglais/publications/AR_2016-2017_EN.pdf

Hema-Quebec, "Annual Report 2017–2018," Available at: www.hema-quebec.qc.ca/userfiles/file/RA2017-2018/RA_2017-2018_EN_2.pdf

Hemphill, Bernice M., "The National Clearinghouse Program of the American Association of Blood Banks," in *Proceedings of Conference on Blood and Blood Banking Drake Hotel, Chicago, December 11–12, 1964* (Chicago: Department of Environmental Health, American Medical Association, 1964): 75–81.

Henry, O., "The Gift of the Magi," in O. Henry, ed., *O'Henry Stories* (New York: Platt & Munk, 1962): 40–48.

Heyman, James, and Dan Ariely, "Effort for Payment: A Tale of Two Markets," *Psychological Science* 15, 11 (2004): 787–793.

Hippen, Benjamin E., *Organ Sales and Moral Travails: Lessons from the Living Kidney Vendor Program in Iran*, Cato Policy Analysis Series, No. 614 (March 20, 2008).

Hoxworth, P.I., Walter E. Haesler, Jr., and Harry Smith, Jr., "The Risk of Hepatitis From Whole Blood and Stored Plasma," *Surgery, Gynecology, & Obstetrics* 109 (1959): 38–42.

Hughes, Paul, "Exploitation, Autonomy, and the Case for Organ Sales," *International Journal of Applied Philosophy* 12, 1 (1998): 89–95.

Iezzoni, Lisa I., Sowmya R. Rao, Catherine M. DesRoches, Christine Vogeli, and Eric G. Campbell, "Survey Shows that at Least Some Physicians are Not Always Open or Honest With Patients," *Health Affairs* 31, 2 (2012): 383–391.

International Society of Blood Transfusion, *A Code Of Ethics For Blood Donation And Transfusion* (2000 amended 2006). Available at: www.isbtweb. org/fileadmin/user_upload/Code_of_Ethics/ISBT_Code_of_Ethics_update_-_feb_2011.pdf.

International Society of Blood Transfusion, "Code of Ethics," Available at: www. ncbi.nlm.nih.gov/pmc/articles/PMC4624526/#b3-blt-13-537

Iorio, Alfonso, Jeffrey S. Stonebraker, Hervé Chambost, Michael Makris, Donna Coffin, Christine Herr, and Federico Germini, "Establishing the Prevalence and Prevalence at Birth of Hemophilia in Males: A Meta-analytic Approach Using National Registries," *Annals of Internal Medicine* 171, 8 (2019): 540–546.

Irlenbusch, Bernd, and Dirk Sliwka, *Incentives, Decision Frames, and Motivation Crowding Out – An Experimental Investigation*, Institute for the Study of Labor IZA DP No. 1758 (September 2005).

Janssen, M.P., L.R. van Hoeven, and G. Rautmann, *Trends and Observations on the Collection, Testing and Use of Blood and Blood Components in Europe 2001–2011 Report* (Strasbourg: European Directorate for the Quality of Medicines & HealthCare of the Council of Europe [EDQM], 2015).

Jasper, J.D., Carol A.E. Nickerson, Peter A. Ubel, David A. Asch, "Altruism, Incentives, and Organ Donation Attitudes of the Transplant Community," *Medical Care* 42, 4 (2004): 378–386.

Jaworski, Peter M., and William English, "The Introduction of Paid Plasma In Canada and the U.S. Has Not Decreased Unpaid Blood Donations," (July 15, 2020): 5. Available at: SSRN: https://ssrn.com/abstract=3653432 or http://dx.doi.org/10.2139/ssrn.3653432

Kant, Immanuel, *The Metaphysics of Morals*, M. Gregor, trans. (Cambridge: Cambridge University Press, 1991).

Kattah, Andrea G., and Vesna D. Garovic, "Preeclampsia: Cardiovascular and Renal Risks During and After Pregnancy," in Babbett LaMarca and Barbara T. Alexander, eds., *Sex Differences in Cardiovascular Physiology and Pathophysiology* (London: Academic Press, 2019): 137–147.

Keown, John, "The Gift of Blood in Europe: An Ethical Defence of EC Directive 89/381," *Journal of Medical Ethics* 23 (1997): 98.

Keown, John, "A reply to McLachlan," *Journal of Medical Ethics* 24 (1998): 255–256.

Kluszczynski, Tomasz, Silvia Rohr, and Rianne Ernst, *White Paper: Key Economic and Value Considerations for Plasma-Derived Medicinal Products (PDMPs) in Europe* (Baarn, The Netherlands: Vintura, 2020), 16.

Koplin, Julian J., "Assessing the Likely Harms to Kidney Vendors in Regulated Organ Markets," *The American Journal of Bioethics* 14, 10 (2014): 7–18.

Koplin, Julian J., "From Blood Donation to Kidney Sales: The Gift Relationship and Transplant Commercialism," *Monash Bioethics Review* 33 (2015): 102–122.

Koplin, Julian J., "Kidney Sales and Market Regulation: A Reply to Semrau," *The Journal of Medicine and Philosophy* 42, 6 (2017): 653–669.

Koplin, Julian J., and Michael J. Selgelid, "The Burden of Proof in Bioethics," *Bioethics* 29, 9 (2015): 597–603.

Koplin, Julian J., and Michael J. Selgelid, "Kidney Sales and the Burden of Proof," *Journal of Practical Ethics* 7, 3 (2019): 32–53.

Kostenzer, Johanna, (on behalf of the EFCNI Working Group on Human Milk Regulation), "Making Human Milk Matter: The Need for EU regulation)," *The Lancet, Child & Adolescent Health* 5, 3 (2021): 161–163.

Kretzmann, Martin J., "Bad Blood: The Moral Stigmatization of Paid Plasma Donors," *Journal of Contemporary Ethnography* 20, 4 (1992): 416–441.

Krever, Horace, *The Commission of Inquiry on the Blood System in Canada – Final Report* (Ottawa, ON: Publications du ministère de la Santé et des Services Sociaux, 1997).

Krishnamurthy, Meena, "Political Solidarity, Justice and Public Health," *Public Health Ethics* 6 (2): 129–141.

Kurlenkova, Alexandra, "Ova Exchange Practises at a Moscow Fertility Clinic: Gift or Commodity?," in Olag Zvonareva, Evgeniya Popova, and Klasien Horstman, eds., *Health, Technologies, and Politics in Post-Soviet Settings* (London: Palgrave MacMillan, 2018): 173–197.

Lacetera, Nicola, "Incentives and Ethics in the Economics of Body Parts," National Bureau of Economic Research Working Paper 22673, 5. Available at: www.nber.org/papers/w22673

Lacetera, Nicola, and Mario Macis, "Time for Blood: The Effect of Paid Leave Legislation on Altruistic Behavior," *The Journal of Law, Economics, and Organization* 29, 6 (2013): 1384–1420.

Lacetera, Nicola, and Mario Macis, "Moral Nimby-Ism? Understanding Societal Support for Monetary Compensation to Plasma Donors in Canada," *Law and Contemporary Problems* 81 (2018): 83–105.

Lacetera, Nicola, Mario Macis, and Robert Slonim, "Will There be Blood? Incentives and Displacement Effects in Pro-Social Behavior," *American Economic Journal* 4, 1 (2012): 186–223.

Lee, Shui Chuen, "Intimacy and Family Consent: A Confucian Ideal," *Journal of Medicine and Philosophy* 40, 4 (2015): 418–436.

Leger, Richard R., "Blood Shortage," *Wall Street Journal* (March 1, 1967).

Locke, John, "Venditio," in Mark Goldie, ed., *Locke: Political Essays* (Cambridge: Cambridge University Press, 1999): 339–343.

Lyons, Daniel, "Welcome Threats and Coercive Offers," *Philosophy* 50, 194 (1975): 425–436.

Maclean, Alasdair, *Autonomy, Informed Consent, and Medical Law: A Relational Challenge* (New York: Cambridge University Press, 2009).

Mahon-Daly, Patricia, "The Alienation of the Gift: The Ethical Use of Donated Blood," *Journal of Medical Law and Ethics* 3, 3 (2015): 193–203.

Maitland, Ian, "The Great Non-Debate Over International Sweatshops," *British Academy of Management Annual Conference Proceedings* (September 1997): 240–265.

Malmqvist, Erik, "Are Bans on Kidney Sales Unjustifiably Paternalistic?" *Bioethics* 28, 3 (2014): 110–118.

Malmqvist, Erik, "Does the Ethical Appropriateness of Paying Donors Depend on What Body Parts They Donate?" *Medicine, Health Care, and Philosophy* 19 (2016): 463–473.

Malootian, Ida, "The 'Emergency' Requisition," in L.P. Holländer, ed., *International Society of Blood Transfusion. 9th Congress, Mexico, September 1962: Proceedings* (Basel: Karger, 1964, vol. 19): 696–699.

Malootian, Ida, "A Plan to Attract Voluntary Blood Donors," in L.P. Holländer, ed., *International Society of Blood Transfusion. 10th Congress, Stockholm, September 1964: Proceedings Part IV: Advances in Blood Transfusion/Treatment of Erythroblastosis Foetalis/Automation/New Equipment/Hepatitis Problems* (Basel: Karger, 1965, vol. 23): 1002–1005.

Marx, Karl, *The Gotha Program* (New York: National Executive Committee Socialist Labor Party, 1922).

McLachlan, Hugh V., "The Unpaid Donation of Blood and Altruism: A Comment on Keown," *Journal of Medical Ethics* 24 (1998): 252–254.

McLean, Sheila A.M., *Autonomy, Consent, and the Law* (New York: Routledge-Cavendish, 2010).

Meisel, Alan, and Loren Roth, "What We Do and Do Not Know about Informed Consent," *Journal of the American Medical Association* 246 (1981): 2473–2477.

Mellstrom, Carl, and Magnus Johannesson, "Crowding Out in Blood Donation: Was Titmuss Right?" *Journal of the European Economic Association* 6, 4 (2008): 845–863.

Meyts, Isabell, Aziz Bousfiha, Carla Duff, Surjit Singh, Yu Lung Lau, Antonio Condino-Neto, Liliana Bezrodnik, Adli Ali, Mehdi Adeli, and Jose Drabwell, "Primary Immunodeficiencies: A Decade of Progress and a Promising Future," *Frontiers in Immunology* 11 (2021): 1–4.

Mill, John Stuart, *On Liberty* (Indianapolis: Hackett Publishing Co., 1978).

Naqvi, Syed Ali Anwar, Bux Ali, Farida Mazhar, Mirza Naqi Zafar, and Syed Adibul Hasan Rizvi, A Socioeconomic Survey of Kidney Vendors in Pakistan," *Transplant International*, 20, 11 (2007): 934–939.

Nathanson v. Klein 350 P2d (1093 Kan 1960).

National Blood Authority, "Why does Australia Import Blood Products?" Available at: www.blood.gov.au/imported-products

National Commission for the Protection of Human Subjects of Biomedical and Behavioral Research, *The Belmont Report* (Washington, DC: DHEW Publication OS 78–0012, 1978).

Noggle, Robert, "Autonomy and the Paradox of Self-Creation: Infinite Regresses, Finite Selves, and the Limits of Authenticity," in James Stacey Taylor, ed., *Personal Autonomy: New Essays on Personal Autonomy and Its Role in Contemporary Moral Philosophy* (Cambridge: Cambridge University Press, 2005): 87–108.

Norris, R.F., "The Carrier of Viral Hepatitis as a Blood Donor," in *Proceedings of the VIIIth Congress of the International Society of Blood Transfusion, 1960* (White Plains, NY: Albert J. Phiebig, Books, 1962): 37–44.

Norris, R.F., "Present Status of Hepatic Function Tests in the Detection of Carriers of Viral Hepatitis," *Paper Presented at IXth International Congress of Society of Blood Transfusion, Mexico City* (September 1962).

Norris, R.F., H. Phelps Potter, Jr., and John G. Reinhold, "Present Status of Hepatic Function Tests in the Detection of Carriers of Viral Hepatitis," *Transfusion* 3, 3 (1963): 202–210.

Octapharma Plasma, "Payments and Rewards," Available at: https://octapharmaplasma.com/donor/payment-rewards

Ontario Public Service Employees Union, "Minutes of the January 25–26 Executive Board Meeting," Available at: https://opseu.org/information/minutes/minutes-of-the-january-25-26-2017-executive-board-meeting/16160/

Oviedo Convention, "Chapter 7, Article 21," Available at: www.coe.int/en/web/conventions/full-list/-/conventions/rms/090000168007cf98

Panitch, Vida, and Lendell Chad Horne, "Paying for Plasma: Commodification, Exploitation, and Canada's Plasma Shortage," *Canadian Journal of Bioethics* 2, 2 (2019): 1–10.

Pellegrino, Edward D., "Patient and Physician Autonomy: Conflicting Rights and Obligations in the Physician-Patient Relationship," *Journal of Contemporary Health Law & Policy* 10, 1 (1994): 47–68.

Penrod, Joshua, and Albert Farrugia, "Errors and Omissions: Donor Compensation Policies and Richard Titmuss," *HEC Forum*, 27, 4 (2015): 319–330.

Penrod, Joshua, and Mary Gustafson, George Schreiber, Jan Bult, and Albert Farrugia, "Response to Volkow P. et al. – Cross-Border Paid Plasma Donation Among Injection Drug Users in Two Mexico – U.S. Border Cities – International Journal of Drug Policy 20 (2009) 409–412," *International Journal of Drug Policy* 21 (2010): 343–344.

Petrini, Carlo, "Production of Plasma-Derived Medicinal Products: Ethical Implications for Blood Donations and Donors," *Blood Transfusion* 12, Supp. 1 (2014): s389–s394.

Pink, J., B. Bell, G. Kotsiou, S. Wright, and J. Thyer, "Safe and Sustainable Plasmapheresis," *ISBT Science Series* 12, 4 (2017): 471–482.

Posner, Richard A., "The Ethics and Economics of Enforcing Contracts of Surrogate Motherhood," *Journal of Contemporary Health Law and Policy* 5 (1989): 21–31.

Potter, Jr., H. Phelps, Norman N. Cohen, and Robert F. Norris, "Chronic Hepatic Dysfunction in Heroin Addicts: Possible Relation to Carrier State of Viral Hepatitis," *Journal of the American Medical Association* 174, 16 (1960): 2049–2051.

Prevot, Johan, and Stephen Jolles, "Global Immunoglobulin Supply: Steaming Towards the Iceberg?" *Current Opinion in Allergy and Clinical Immunology* 20, 6 (2020): 557–564.

Pricop, Laura, "Blood and Plasma Donors During the COVID-19 Pandemic: Arguments Against Financial Stimulation," *History and Philosophy of the Life Sciences* 43, Article 29 (2021). Available at: https://doi.org/10.1007/s40656-021-00389-4

Protein Plasma Therapeutics Association, "IQPP Qualified Donor Standard Version 4.0," (June 25, 2014). Available at: www.pptaglobal.org/images/IQPP/QualifiedDonorStdFinal1.pdf

Protein Plasma Therapeutics Association, "Plasma Protein Therapies," Available at: www.pptaglobal.org/plasma-protein-therapies

Protein Plasma Therapeutics Association, "Updated Response to Ontario's Proposal to Ban Compensated Plasma Donation," Available at: www.pptaglobal.org/membership/current-members/28-news/ppta-news/900-ppta-s-updated-response-to-ontario-s-proposal-to-ban-compensated-plasma-donation

Protein Plasma Therapeutics Association, "What is Plasma?" Available at: www.pptaglobal.org/plasma

Province of Alberta, "Voluntary Blood Donations Act," Assented to (March 30, 2017). Available at: www.qp.alberta.ca/documents/Acts/V05.pdf

Province of Alberta, "Voluntary Blood Donations Repeal Act," Assented to (December 9, 2020). Available at: www.qp.alberta.ca/Documents/AnnualVolumes/2020/ch41_2020.pdf

Province of British Columbia, "Voluntary Blood Donations Act," Assented to (May 31, 2018). Available at: www.bclaws.ca/civix/document/id/lc/statreg/18030

Puyol, Angel, "Ética, Solidaridad y Donación de Sangre. Cuatro perspectivas para debater," *Revista de Bioetica Derecho* 45 (2019): 44–58.

Radcliffe Richards, Janet, *The Ethics of Transplants: Why Careless Thought Costs Lives* (Oxford: Oxford University Press, 2012).

Radcliffe Richards, Janet, "Not a Defence of Organ Markets," *Journal of Practical Ethics* 7, 3 (2019): 54–66.

Radin, Margaret Jane, *Contested Commodities* (Cambridge, MA: Harvard University Press, 1996).

Raz, Joseph, *The Morality of Freedom* (Oxford: Clarendon Press, 1986).

Read, Leonard E., *I, Pencil* (Atlanta, GA: Foundation for Economic Education, 2019).

Rebanks, James, *The Shepherd's Life: A tale of the Lake District* (London: Allen Lane, 2015).

Reddy Snigdha, and Belinda Jim, "Hypertension and Pregnancy: Management and Future Risks," *Advances in Chronic Kidney Disease* 26, 2 (2019): 137–145.

Ricardo, David, *On the Principles of Political Economy and Taxation* (London: J. M. Dent & Sons, 1911).

Roback, John D., and Jeanette Guarner, "Convalescent Plasma to Treat COVID-19: Possibilities and Challenges," *Journal of the American Medical Association* 323, 16 (2020): 1561–1562.

Robert, Patrick, "Self-sufficiency: Facts and Pitfalls!" *The Source* (Fall 2014): 32–38.

Rodell, M., "Collection of Source Material From Remunerated Donors," *Developments in Biological Standardization* 81 (1993): 57–64.

Rodell, M.B., and M.L. Lee, "Determination of Reasons for Cessation of Participation in Serial Plasmapheresis Programs," *Transfusion* 39 (1999): 900–903.

Rossi, Françoise, "The Organization of Transfusion and Fractionation in France and Its Regulation," *Annals of Blood* 3 (2018). Available at: http://aob.amegroups.com/article/view/4610/5358

Rovira, Ll. Puig, "Plasma Self-Sufficiency in Spain," *Transfusion and Apheresis Science* 59, 1 (2020): 2. Available at: https://doi.org/10.1016/j.transci.2019.102700

Sandel, Michael J., *What Money Can't Buy: The Moral Limits of Markets* (New York: Farrar, Straus and Giroux, 2012).

Schneider, T., O. Fontaine, and J.J. Huart, "Éthiques, motivations des donneurs d'aphérèse plasmatique," *Transfusion Clinique et Biologique* 11, 3 (2004): 146–152.

Schreiber, George B., Roger Brinser, Marilyn Rosa-Bray, Zi-Fan Yu, and Toby Simon, "Frequent Source Plasma Donors are not at Risk of Iron Depletion: The Ferritin Levels in Plasma Donor (FLIPD) Study," *Transfusion* 58 (2018): 951–959.

Schreiber, George B., and Mary Clare Kimber, "Source Plasma Donors: A Snapshot," *Poster Presented AABB Annual Meeting, San Diego, CA* (October 7–10, 2017). Available at: www.pptaglobal.org/images/presentations/2017/Schreiber. AABBposterAbstract_Source_Plasma_Donors_A_Snapshot_2017_9.27.17.pdf

Schulzki, T., K. Seidel, H. Storch, H. Karges, S. Kiessig, S. Schneider, U. Taborski, K. Wolter, D. Steppat, E. Behm, M. Zeisner, and P. Hellstern for the SIPLA study group, "A Prospective Multicentre Study on the Safety of Long-Term Intensive Plasmapheresis in Donors (SIPLA)," *Vox Sanguinis* 91 (2006): 162–173.

Schwartz, Gary T., "The Myth of the Ford Pinto Case," *Rutgers Law Review* 43 (1991): 1013–1068.

Schwartz, Joel, "Blood and Altruism," *Public Interest* 136 (1999): 35–51.

Shaffer, H. Luke, and Analidis Ochoa, "How Blood-Plasma Companies Target the Poorest Americans," *The Atlantic* (March 15, 2018).

Shahed, Kazi Safowan, Abdullahil Azeem, Syed Mithun Ali, and Md. Abdul Moktadir, "A Supply Chain Disruption Risk Mitigation Model to Manage COVID-19 Pandemic Risk," *Environmental Science and Pollution Research* (January 15, 2021). Available at: https://doi.org/10.1007/s11356-020-12289-4

Shaz, Beth H., Ronald E. Domen, and Christopher R. France, "Remunerating Donors to Ensure a Safe and Available Blood Supply," *Transfusion* 60, S3 (2020): S134–S137.

Shearmur, Jeremy, "Trust, Titmuss, and Blood," *Economic Affairs* 21, 1 (2001): 29–33.

Singer, Peter, "Altruism and Commerce: A Defense of Titmuss against Arrow," *Philosophy & Public Affairs* 2, 3 (1973): 312–320.

Skey, Michael, "Why Do Nations Matter? The Struggle for Belonging and Security in an Uncertain World," *The British Journal of Sociology* 64, 1 (2013): 81–98.

Skinner, M.W., P. Ann Hedlund Hoppe, Henry G. Grabowski, Richard Manning, Raffi Tachdjian, James F. Crone, and Stuart J. Youngner, "Risk-Based Decision Making and Ethical Considerations in Donor Compensation for Plasma-Derived Medicinal Products," *Transfusion* 56, 11 (2016): 2889–2894.

Slonim, Robert, Carmen Wang, and Ellen Garbarino, "The Market for Blood," *Journal of Economic Perspectives* 28, 2 (2014): 177–196.

Smith, Adam, *An Inquiry into the Nature and Causes of the Wealth of Nations* (Chicago: University of Chicago Press, 1976).

Smith, II, George P., "Through a Test Tube Darkly: Artificial Insemination and the Law," *Michigan Law Review* 67, 1 (1968): 127–150.

Staff author, "Blood Money," *Medical World News* (March 15, 1963): 136.

Staff author, "No Fun in This Joint," *Medical World News* (March 15, 1963): 136.

Staff author, "Yes, We've Some Bananas," *Medical World News* (March 15, 1963): 136.

Steinhardt, Bernice, *Enhancing Safeguards Would Strengthen the Nation's Blood Supply* (Washington, DC: United States General Accounting Office, June 5, 1997).

Strengers, Paul F.W., "Evidence-Based Clinical Indications of Plasma Products and Future Prospects," *Annals of Blood* 2, 9 (2017): 1–7.

Strengers, Paul F.W., and Harvey G. Klein, "Plasma is a Strategic Resource," *Transfusion* 56, 12 (2016): 3133–3137.

Tabor, E., "The Epidemiology of Virus Transmission by Plasma Derivatives: Clinical Studies Verifying the Lack of Transmission of Hepatitis B and C viruses and HIV Type 1," *Transfusion* 39 (1999): 1160–1168.

Taylor, James Stacey, "Autonomy, Duress, and Coercion," *Social Philosophy & Policy* 20, 2 (2003): 127–155.

Taylor, James Stacey, "Autonomy and Informed Consent: A Much Misunderstood Relationship," *Journal of Value Inquiry*, 38, 3 (2004): 383–391.

Taylor, James Stacey, *Stakes and Kidneys: Why Markets in Human Body Parts are Morally Imperative* (Aldershot, UK: Ashgate, 2005).

Taylor, James Stacey, "Kidney Problems," *The Times Higher Education Supplement* (April 14, 2006). Available at: www.timeshighereducation.com/com ment/letters/kidney-problems/202593.article

Taylor, James Stacey, "Introduction," in *Personal Autonomy: New Essays on Personal Autonomy and Its Role in Contemporary Moral Philosophy* (Cambridge: Cambridge University Press, 2008): 1–31.

Taylor, James Stacey, *Practical Autonomy and Bioethics* (New York: Routledge, 2009).

Taylor, James Stacey, *Death, Posthumous Harm, and Bioethics* (New York: Routledge, 2012).

Taylor, James Stacey, "A Scandal in Geneva: Culpable Negligence and the WHO's 2013 Report on National Self-Sufficiency in Blood and Blood Products," *International Journal of Applied Philosophy* 28, 2 (2014): 219–234.

Taylor, James Stacey, "Why Policies that Aim at National Self-Sufficiency in Blood and Blood Products are (Usually) Unethical," *Public Affairs Quarterly* 29, 3 (2015): 313–326.

Taylor, James Stacey, "WTF WHO?" *HEC Forum* 27 (2015): 287–300.

Taylor, James Stacey, "How Not to Argue for Markets, or, Why the Argument from Mutually Beneficial Exchange Fails," *Journal of Social Philosophy* 48, 2 (2017): 165–179.

Taylor, James Stacey, "Why Prohibiting Donor Compensation Can Prevent Plasma Donors from Giving Their Informed Consent to Donate," *Journal of Medicine and Philosophy*, 44, 1 (2019): 10–32.

Taylor, James Stacey, "The Ethics and Politics of Blood Plasma Donation: The Case in Canada," *International Journal of Applied Philosophy* 34, 1 (2020): 89–103.

Taylor, James Stacey, *Markets with Limits: How the Commodification of Academia Derails Debate* (New York: Routledge, forthcoming).

Tehran, Hoda Ahmari, Shohreh Tashi, Nahid Mehran, Narges Eskandari, and Tahmineh Dadkhah Tehrani, "Emotional Experiences in Surrogate Mothers: A Qualitative Study," *Iranian Journal of Reproductive Medicine* 12, 7 (2014): 471–480.

Thalberg, Irving, "Hierarchical Analyses of Unfree Action," *Canadian Journal of Philosophy* 8, 2 (1978): 211–226.

Thorpe, Rachel, Barbara M. Masser, Kyle Jensen, Nina Van Dyke, and Tanya E. Davison, "The Role of Identity in How Whole-Blood Donors Reflect on and Construct Their Future as a Plasma Donor," *Journal of Community & Applied Social Psychology* 30, 1 (2020): 73–84.

Titmuss, Richard M., *The Gift Relationship: From Human Blood to Social Policy* (New York: Vintage Books, 1971).

Tobin, James, "On Limiting the Domain of Inequality," *Journal of Law and Economics* 13, 2 (1970): 263–277.

Trimmelm, Michael, Helene Lattacher, and Monika Janda, "Voluntary Whole-Blood Donors, and Compensated Platelet Donors and Plasma Donors: Motivation to Donate, Altruism and Aggression," *Transfusion and Apheresis Science* 33 (2005): 147–155.

United Kingdom Government, Department of Health and Social Care, "Ban Lifted to Allow UK Blood Plasma to be Used for Life-Saving Treatments," (February 25, 2021). Available at: www.gov.uk/government/news/ban-lifted-to-allow-uk-blood-plasma-to-be-used-for-life-saving-treatments

United States Census Bureau (CB12–255), Available at: www.census.gov/news room/releases/archives/population/cb12-255.html

United States General Accounting Office, "Plasma Product Risks Are Low if Good Manufacturing Practices are Followed," *Report to the Chairman, Subcommittee on Human Resources, Committee on Government Reform and Oversight, House of Representatives* (September 9, 1998). Available at: www.gao.gov/assets/hehs-98-205.pdf (Accessed March 29, 2021).

United States Government National Highway Traffic Safety Administration, Available at: www.nhtsa.gov/vehicle/2015/FORD/FUSION/4%252520DR/FWD

Veldhuizen, Ingrid, and Anne van Dongen, "Motivational Differences Between Whole Blood and Plasma Donors Already Exist before Their First Donation Experience," *Transfusion* 58, 3 (2012): 1678–1686.

Volkow, P., et al., "Cross-Border Paid Plasma Donation Among Injection Drug Users in Two Mexico – U.S. Border Cities," *International Journal of Drug Policy* 20, 5 (2009): 409–412.

Waldby, Catherine, and Robert Mitchell. *Tissue Economies: Blood, Organs, and Cell Lines* (Durham, NC: Duke University Press, 2008).

Walsh, Adrian, "Compensation for Blood Plasma Donation as a *Distinctive* Ethical Hazard: Reformulating the Commodification Objection," *HEC Forum* 27, 4 (2015): 401–416.

Warneken, Felix, and Michael Tomasello, "Extrinsic Rewards Undermine Altruistic Tendencies in 20-Month-Olds," *Developmental Psychology* 44, 6 (2008): 1785–1788.

Warnock, Mary, "Will Liberty Lead us to an Internal Market?" *The Times Higher Education Supplement* (April 7, 2006). Available at: www.timeshigher education.com/books/will-liberty-lead-us-to-an-internal-market/202438.article

Weidmanna, Christian, Sven Schneider, Eberhard Weck, Dagmar Menzel, Harald Klüter, and Michael Müller-Steinhardt, "Monetary Compensation and Blood Donor Return: Results of a Donor Survey in Southwest Germany," *Transfusion Medicine and Hemotherapy* 41 (2014): 257–262.

Weimer, Steven, "'I Can't Eat if I Don't Plass': Impoverished Plasma Donors, Alternatives, and Autonomy," *HEC Forum* 27 (2015): 261–285.

Weinstein, Mark, "Regulation of Plasma for Fractionation in the United States," *Annals of Blood* 2, 3 (2018): 1–15.

Wertheimer, Alan, *Exploitation* (Princeton: Princeton University Press, 1996).

Wheeler, Jr., Charles B., "State Laws and Regulations," in *Proceedings of Conference on Blood and Blood Banking Drake Hotel, Chicago, December 11–12, 1964* (Chicago: Department of Environmental Health, American Medical Association, 1964): 122–128.

White, Amy E., "The Morality of an Internet Market in Human Ova," *Journal of Value Inquiry* 40 (2006): 311–321.

White, Lucie, "Does Remuneration for Plasma Compromise Autonomy?," *HEC Forum* 27 (2015): 387–400.

WHO Expert Group, "Expert Consensus Statement on Achieving Self-Sufficiency in Safe Blood and Blood Products Based on Voluntary Non-Remunerated Blood Donation (VNRBD)," *Vox Sanguinis* 103, 4 (2012): 337–342.

Wilkinson, Stephen, *Bodies for Sale: Ethics and Exploitation in the Human Body Trade* (New York: Routledge, 2003).

Wilkinson, Stephen, "The Exploitation Argument Against Commercial Surrogacy," *Bioethics* 17, 2 (2003): 169–187.

Wilkinson, T.M., *Ethics and the Acquisition of Organs* (Oxford: Oxford University Press, 2011).

Williams, Alan E., "FDA Considerations Regarding Frequent Plasma Collection Procedures," *15th International Haemovigilance Seminar, Brussels, Belgium.* Available at: www.ihn-org.com/wp-content/

Wood, Allen, "Exploitation," *Social Philosophy & Policy* 12 (1995): 136–158.

World Health Assembly, "Sixty-Third World Health Assembly, Resolution WHA63.12," Available at: http://apps.who.int/gb/ebwha/pdf_files/WHA63/A63_R12-en.pdf

World Health Organization, *Towards Self-Sufficiency in Safe Blood and Blood Products based on Voluntary Non-remunerated Donation* (Geneva: World Health Organization, 2013).

World Health Organization, *2016 Global Status Report on Blood Safety and Availability* (Geneva: WHO, 2017).

World Health Organization, *World Health Organization Model List of Essential Medicines, 21st List, 2019* (Geneva: World Health Organization, 2019. Licence: CC BY-NC-SA 3.0 IGO).

World Health Organization, "Blood Safety and Availability," Available at: www.who.int/mediacentre/factsheets/fs279/en/index.html

World Health Organization, "The Rome Declaration on Achieving Self-Sufficiency in Safe Blood and Blood Products, based on Voluntary Non-Remunerated Donation," Available at: www.avis.it/userfiles/file/RomeDeclarationSelf-SufficiencySafeBloodBloodProductsVNRD.pdf

Young, Robert, "The Value of Autonomy," *The Philosophical Quarterly* 32, 126 (1982): 35–44.

Ythier, J. Mercier, "The Contested Market of Plasma," *Transfusion Clinique et Biologique* 27, 1 (2020): 52–57.

Zimmerman, David, "Coercive Wage Offers," *Philosophy & Public Affairs* 10, 2 (1981): 121–145.

Zwolinski, Matt, "The Ethics of Price Gouging," *Business Ethics Quarterly* 18, 3 (2008): 347–378.

Index

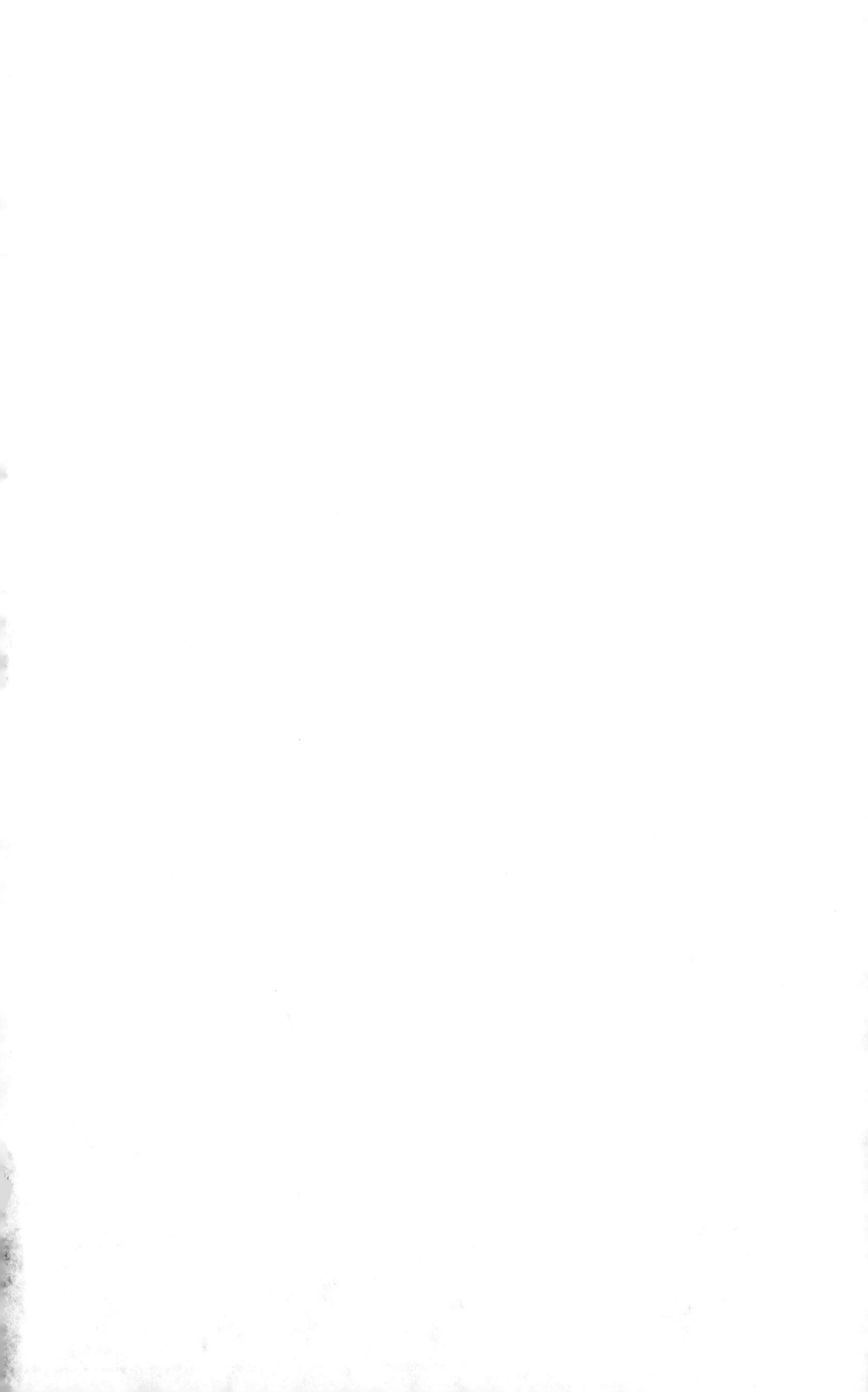

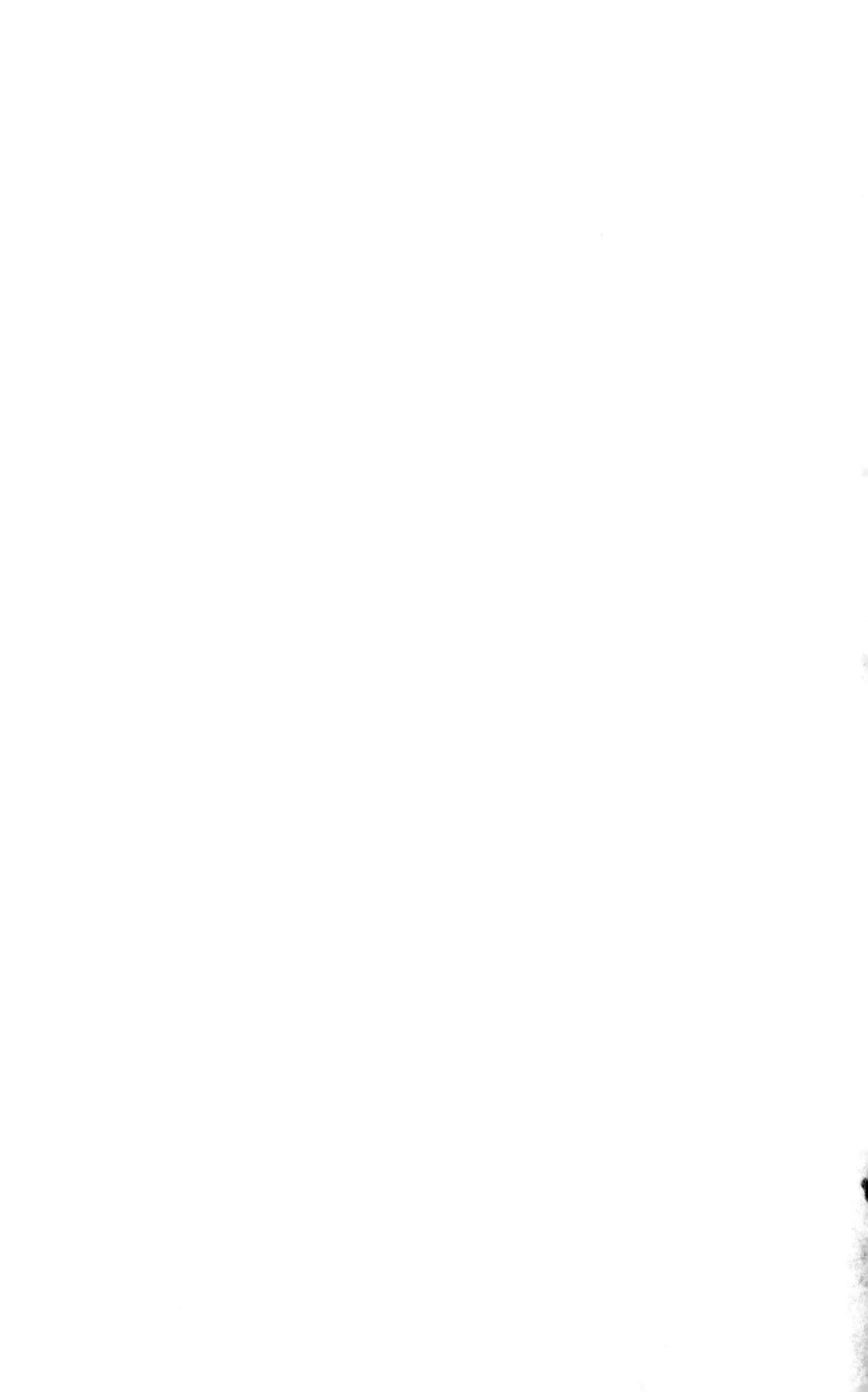